Book Description

Your body is not meant to thrive if you are constantly eating. Yes, you read that right. Have you been struggling with health issues for years despite trying everything? There's a simple reason for that. Our ancestors were hunter-gatherers, surviving in a fast-feast cycle. They had to go for long periods without food. In response to these conditions, the human body developed the *thrifty gene*. In those days, this gene had real functionality. Its job was to store nutrients for when the body would go through periods of food shortage. So, it ensured that even if you had to go for days without food, you still had enough energy to get by.

Time passed, technology took over, and now here we are. Most of us have no use for the *thrifty gene* anymore. Food is available for consumption at a hand's reach. And for some of us, eating healthy means eating regularly spaced out meals all through the day.

What if I told you this is wrong? That your body will do better if allowed to rest between periods of eating? That it will finally be able to tap into your fat reserves instead of glucose and use that to burn energy, therefore making you healthier, fitter, and younger?

This book will be your roadmap in understanding the a to z of intermittent fasting. Backed by the words of experts in the field, intermittent fasting is here to revolutionize the very way in which you eat. Simply speaking, it is a schedule of eating where you alternate your regular calorie intake with lesser or zero-calorie intake days. The book will take you through a detailed explanation of what it is, its types and their characteristics, finding your fit, and even give you an idea of what the internet thinks! Most importantly, you will learn the science behind intermittent fasting and why it is more effective as a fat-burning tool than many other approaches, including a ketogenic diet. You will learn about its far-reaching effects on weight loss and for improving insulin sensitivity, brain health, and heart health; healing inflammation; and fighting cancer and anti-aging.

Years back, Benjamin Franklin said, *"The best medicines are resting and fasting."* Little did we know how correct he was. Welcome to your future.

Intermittent Fasting for a Healthier You

A Guide to Reset Your Metabolism, Supercharge your Energy, Speed Up Weight Loss and Detox your Body

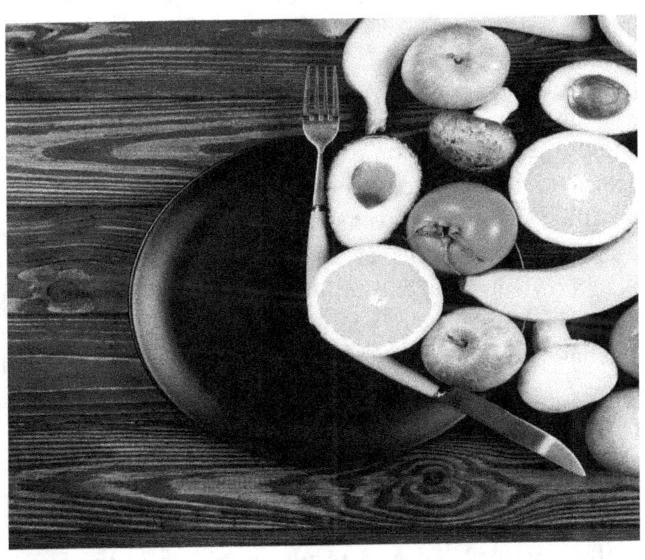

Shawnie Perez

Table of Contents

Introduction: Georgie gets a Key — 1

Chapter 1: Intermittent Fasting: What Is It? — 7

  Understanding Our Bodies — 8

  History and Terminology — 13

Chapter 2: Alexa, What Does the Internet Say? — 21

Chapter 3: Types, Assets, Drawbacks — 26

  The Twice-a-Week Approach — 26

  The Alternate Day Fast — 29

  Time-Restricted Feeding — 32

    A Note on Liquid Consumption — 36

Chapter 4: Weight Loss, Diabetes, and Intermittent Fasting — 38

  Weight Loss — 38

  Insulin Sensitivity and Diabetes Control — 40

Chapter 5: Autophagy and Cancer — 44

  Inflammation — 48

Chapter 6: Cardiovascular Health, Brain Function, and Anti-Aging — 51

  Cardiovascular Health — 51

  Brain Health — 53

  Anti-Aging Properties — 55

    Tips to Get You Started — 57

      Who should think twice before attempting intermittent fasting? — 59

Chapter 7: Success Stories — 61

  Jennie Turns Her Life Around — 61

  Naomi Gets Another Chance — 65

  57 Years Young — 69

Chapter 8: A Day of Meals with Me!   72

  Brunch   72

  3 pm Meal   73

  Dinner   74

    Dessert   75

Conclusion: My Story   78

References   81

Introduction: Georgie gets a Key

For the majority of her 27 years, Georgie and health-issues were the best of friends. She was notorious in her circles for her horrible relationship with her stomach. Not that she never tried to fix things. She tried everything, from cutting out oil and spice, heavy carbohydrates, to several ill-fated vegetables which did nothing for her weight-loss. She went to countless doctors and tried new diets, harder workouts, and gastric pills. When the heartburn would come, however, she would feel physically incapacitated. It would creep up her body as if moving to her lungs, spread through her hands, and make its way to her mind. She would be bed-ridden for days on end. She stopped eating out altogether and took recourse to purging her meals for fear of more pain. Nothing helped. As her food sensitivity grew, so did her anxiety, to the extent that she felt completely powerless over her own life choices. Everything she did was dictated by what she would eat, the timings, and the subsequent effects. Food became the monster under the bed. No matter how hard she tried, she could not rid herself of the obsession until she heard of two magic words: intermittent fasting.

Georgie knew to do her research before she began. Years of failed diets and emerging health problems had taught her to cross-check everything. She found that intermittent fasting had garnered a great deal of positive attention over the years. Its advocates promised lasting weight loss, reduction of body fat, increasing health, motivation, and cognitive development, and a whole new approach to life marked by immense willpower and positivity. Georgie consulted a dietician and made a plan for herself. She put her mind, body, and soul into practicing intermittent fasting for two years. She hasn't looked back since.

Research told her that Time-restricted Eating (TRE) resulted in several health benefits, which included the betterment of heart function and increased aerobic capacity, without requiring one to change their diet. That meant that she could eat the same food in the same quantity, simply within a 'restricted' time frame. She found that finishing her meals within the time frame of six hours reduced her appetite, made her feel more energetic, and gave her a whole week without gastric influx.

Georgie was grateful for the simple nature of her new routine. She did not have to make a whole new diet plan including complex supplements or expensive food items. She didn't even have to think of new meal plans or worry about what to cook for herself the moment she woke up. The very thought of that had given her nightmares for years. Now, she would wake up and get on with her day, beginning her six-hour eating frame at noon and finishing by six in the evening. Not only did this increase her energy over time, but she also found herself looking forward to every day. Life was becoming an adventure. She woke up with a clean stomach and she went to bed feeling just right. She could go for longer runs without worrying about her heart giving out. She went out with her friends, ate popcorn in the movies, and even managed to lunch at restaurants once in a while! She found that 90 percent of her life had been spent making decisions about what to cook for breakfast and dinner. Now, she felt free from that burden, from the anxiety of always choosing wrong. Her willpower returned, stronger than ever before. The first few months were the hardest because when one is adjusting one's body to a new schedule, fatigue is always a given. Yet, the more she progressed, the more her body became strong, her skin glowed, and she felt empowered. Discipline, once inculcated, is a valuable trait. Georgie found that the invisible arms that food wrapped so tightly around her were finally loosening, and the more they loosened, the more she took flight.

At first, she thought she would not make it. Her work ended at five, and she came home to a meal. She always liked to eat later in the day so that she would not get hungry, and now, she found herself waking up at midnight with a rumbling stomach. She missed her Coffee-Mate in the morning. The notion of fitting in all of her calories from the course of a whole day to a six-hour time frame challenged her, pushed her, and finally, disciplined her. The other benefits that followed were additional and most welcome. Georgie had more energy and time for workouts.

Georgie did not begin intermittent fasting to lose weight. She just wanted to get better. As time passed, she also noted immense physical progress. For her, this was very uplifting. She was no stranger to exercise, but for the last few years, her workouts had not provided any results except taking her to a stage of physical depletion where she was too tired to feel sad or alone. Fasting brought about a huge change. She became more toned and found her workouts becoming easier and more enjoyable. The anger with which she approached life was becoming replaced with hope. She found the energy to try new workouts, go hiking, and even take on the invites from her friends for a round of spin class and yoga.

Georgie's life did a 180-degree turn in the year that she began practicing intermittent fasting. Have you felt like Georgie? You can be at any phase in your life and still be crippled by your eating habits. I know of nothing worse than waking up to the dread of planning your next meal and wondering if it will cause you any pain.

At a personal level, I have lived with an eating disorder for years. My eating habits went out of control when I was a young adult, trying to shape my body by the dictates imposed on me by society, my peers, and most importantly, my own unrealistic expectations. I would binge and purge for days, go without food for days, and I would exercise for five hours at a stretch and deplete myself until I just did not have the energy to think about food anymore. My dear reader, do not let this be your life. Food is so precious; it is so nourishing. It is fuel to your body and mind, and if done correctly, eating is one of the greatest pleasures and privileges that are given to mankind. You have it in you to control your body and to take it to a point where it becomes a vehicle for you to enjoy your life. I'm going to pause here to draw on a few scientific studies.

In 2018, a research report published by Nutrition and Healthy Aging discussed a study where 23 individuals practiced intermittent fasting for 12 weeks. They consumed their meals within an eight-hour timeframe, and following the twelve weeks, researchers compared their weight loss results to another control group. The results of the former group showed a three percent greater loss in weight, on average. Additionally, there was a reduction in blood pressure among the participants (Kristin et al., 2018).

We will discuss scientific research later in this book. For now, I want to focus on you. How tired are you of living a life which always has you feeling out-of-control? When I was in the deep with my eating disorder, I spent 13 hours a day simply planning meals. Not the hopeful planning that one does in the expectation of good results. I was obsessed. I could not think beyond the burger for lunch, the acidity that would follow, the ice-cream here, and the fries and ketchup there. Unhealthy eating became my mantra, and the more it made me sick, the more I obsessed with it. I needed the pain in my life. I put myself through an endless trip of junk food, guilt, more junk food, purge, and repeat. I had no urge to eat healthy because it felt like such a waste of time. Eating healthy brought no results, I had no energy for exercise and I made excuses so that I would not have to step outside my house or meet anyone else. I just wanted to hide within my four walls, crying over tubs of cheese popcorn and bars of chocolate. Needless to say, my life was in desperate need of a glow-up.

When I encountered intermittent fasting, I took it up more as a last resort. My chest pains had gotten so bad I felt

I would be hospitalized from the sheer sleeplessness they brought me. I could not breathe on some days, I could not walk, and I could not even get up without feeling like I would collapse. Crazy, right? All this just from gastric issues! The thing is, our body is the sum total of component parts, and when you begin abusing one part repeatedly, everything else eventually falls apart. Intermittent fasting took me through a rough ride at first. I was so used to the irregularity of my meals and just eating whatever I wanted whenever I wanted to that I could not make my body understand, "It's six pm, no more food for you!" The only reason I pushed through was the desire to truly change. At the two-month mark, changes started happening. I was no longer hungry. I had the urge to do better and to be better. I started looking forward to planning my meals and to actually enjoying them!

This book is a labor of love. I have suffered the negative implications of a poor diet for years. When I began intermittent fasting, it was a decision to give my body the kindness it deserved. It feels personal to me. I have walked a long road, and I want to take you on that journey too. If you have this in front of you, you are someone looking to change your life for the better. I truly hope this book will be a key in your hands, pushing you to open the door to the life which is waiting for you.

Chapter 1: Intermittent Fasting: What Is It?

The health and fitness industry has been in the throes of a curious dichotomy for the last few years. On the one hand, there has been increased growth in the popularity of fad diets, programs promising results in a week, and stringent weight measurement plans, all based on little or no research. On the other hand, obesity has also been on the rise, with the easy availability of fast-food chains, more and more office hours requiring long hours in front of a desktop, easy access to entertainment, and growing dependence on take-outs and armchair comfort (Ganesan et al., 2018). A report published by the World Health Organization in 2016 marked over 1.9 billion overweight and over 650 million obese people worldwide, triple the numbers from a study in 1975. Obesity is the starting point of several metabolic disorders, like coronary heart diseases, cancer, osteoarthritis, and bad respiratory health. A meta-analysis done by Galani and Schneider in 2007 advocates for lifestyle changes to reduce weight and the overall propensity for cardiovascular diseases (Galani & Schneider, 2007). According to their study, lifestyle interventions have been proven to cause improvements in metabolic aberrations. These programs function like interventions, focusing on aspects such as a healthy lifestyle, regulated eating patterns, dietary counseling, and a new approach to the way we eat[1].

The take-away from this is that lifestyle changes are the only long-term road to a healthy life. There are no fad diets, crash courses lasting seven days, or starve-yourself-to-fit body programs that will allow for your physical and mental well-being in the long run. You may think that it doesn't matter as long as you see results now, but also think— two years from now, all the effort you have put in amounts to nothing and you are back right where you started. That doesn't sound promising, does it? Which brings us to the next question— what is intermittent fasting and why is it a lifestyle change? We don't usually associate the term 'fasting' with anything long-term, so how is this any different?

Understanding Our Bodies

Your body is home to millions of cells. Every cell is self-contained. Each of them represents an individual

---

[1] Galani's study based itself on a systematic review of the literature available on restrictive eating. The study included randomized clinical trials (topic lifestyle intervention) of overweight/obese subjects during a minimum of a one-year period. It evaluated outcomes based on body weight, blood lipid, glucose control, fasting plasma glucose, two-hour plasma glucose, high and low-density lipoprotein, and glycosylated hemoglobin. It chose 13 reports on the prevention and 17 on the treatment of obesity. It was found that, placed against standard care, lifestyle intervention was significantly more effective in reducing body pressure, blood lipids, and blood glucose of the subjects. These reductions were maintained up to a three-year period (Galani & Schneider, 2007).

living entity. Just as we keep like-minded people close, the cells of the same type like to join together. They use intercellular substances to establish this communication. As a result, human tissues, like muscles, are formed. When tissues join together, they create our organs. At a higher level, several organs cooperate to get work done. For instance, your digestive system is the result of functions of organs that begin straight at the mouth and reach your colon. The whole body is a living, thriving machine composed of parts that help each other in helping you to exist.

Your organs contribute to your overall health and state of being. In return, your health influences how effectively your organs function. Your cells are in a constant state of function, engaging in chemical reactions to keep up with the production of new substances and the breakdown of old ones. For example, the bones in your body are made of tissues that break down and regenerate for the first few decades of your life. So, just like we need the energy to work, the cells need it to do the same. Cells require energy in the forms of carbohydrates, protein, and fat. All of these produce energy, which is used at different levels depending on availability. Your body is programmed to use carbohydrates before moving to protein or fat utilization for energy. The cells also need water, minerals, vitamins, and oxygen. All of these enable proper tissue function. So, broadly speaking, we can refer to carbohydrates, proteins, fats, vitamins, minerals, oxygen, and every other item your body needs to survive as enablers. These enablers are your nutrients. They are responsible for nourishment.

This is where all of us must agree on one thing: simply eating food will not nourish you. Your body has to work at digesting the food and make it into usable components that can be absorbed by your bloodstream. Without this process, the food you eat will not be available for use by cells. Our actions are mostly involuntary. None of us will pause to think that the burger we are enjoying will enter our bodies and blood systems in a completely different form than when it enters our mouths. So, in a way, our bodies know what to do for us. You do not need to sit down and give a lecture to your cells about why they should absorb the last meal you ate. Your body will find a way to do that without your instructions. You do not consciously decide that your pancreas will aid digestion, how quickly the food you eat will be absorbed, or when a sugar-rush will hit you. At every step, your body is deciding for you.

The food you eat does not immediately become nutrients. It goes through stages of ingestion, digestion, propulsion, and finally, absorption. The elements which do not get absorbed go through a natural elimination process. The whole digestion process happens in your gastrointestinal tract with some help from other organs. This tract is the combination of your mouth, pharynx, esophagus, stomach, small and large intestine, and anus. Your gastrointestinal tract has sphincters that regulate the proper flow of food particles. Muscle contractions enable this flow. Nerves and hormones enable these muscle contractions. So, you see, every process is connected to the next.

Metabolism is the key to all the chemical processes that happen in your body. It regulates your life. The whole sequence of chemical reactions performed by your body cells comprises metabolism. The cell cytoplasm and organelles release and use energy from the food you eat, synthesizing useful energy and deciding what needs to be excreted. Metabolism functions via two reactions. The first is anabolic, which puts different molecules together, therefore requiring lots of energy. The second is catabolic, which takes molecules apart and releases energy. Carbohydrates, proteins, and fats (macronutrients) work to give energy, while vitamins and minerals (micronutrients) contribute to enzyme activities that encourage metabolic reactions in your cells. The process of energy production begins in the cytoplasm, where glucose is broken down. Other aerobic actions happen in the mitochondria. The sum of all these processes leads to a breakdown of energy in food to energy stored in the compound adenosine triphosphate. This is the cell's energy currency. Whatever movement of energy happens, happens via this.

Now, who would think of so much when they eat? Given how immediate human needs for gratification have become, all of us mainly eat to satisfy hunger. The problems happen when other things come into play. In the current context, hunger is not the only reason we ingest food. We eat at social gatherings, when we are depressed, when we are bored, or simply because we need something to munch on while our favorite television show is on. The food habits of any society rely on the overall cultural, social, economic, and psychological environment. A big problem in many contemporary societies is how to strike a balance between energy intake and expenditure. When the intake far exceeds expenditure, excess calories deposit in your body as fat stores. The body has no use for them but decides to keep them around, just in case— a safety deposit, if you will.

Providing adequate nutrition to your body is the key to a long, healthy life. When you are thinking of providing nutrition, you have to go beyond the obvious ingestion of calories. Timing is just as important. Understanding when your body needs food and when it can do without is one of the most important realizations you will come to. As I mentioned before, your body does not need you to tell it to burn calories for energy. It will do so itself. Sometimes, it may even trick you into thinking that it needs you to consume food, even if there is enough energy supply to tap from.

The more fat builds up in your body, the more health implications. Skinny people can also face the consequences of this. Yes, you heard that right. Many of us have what nutritionists like to call "skinny fat," which is also a risk factor for obesity, type 2 diabetes, and other cardiovascular diseases. It is an indication that your body doesn't have enough lean muscle and is carrying excess visceral fat. Visceral fat envelops crucial organs of your body like the liver, kidneys, and intestine. Too much of it and the proper function of all of these organs are impacted negatively.

In the following chapters, we will learn about intermittent fasting and how it helps your body find balance. If you give your body the chance to use the deposits you have made over the years, weight loss and health benefits will follow. If you have struggled with maintaining a diet and exercise isn't helping as it should, intermittent fasting may give you the push you need. Your liver can hold approximately 700 calories of glucose. During the fasting period, you are pushing your liver to burn this. This will take about 12 hours and then be followed by a metabolic switch. And voila, your body will turn to fat for energy. Does this sound exciting to you? Then let's get into the history and science behind intermittent fasting.

History and Terminology

Studies on the application of intermittent fasts for treating obesity date back to the early 20th century. Many of these early studies were based on short-term starvation periods ranging from one to fourteen days. For instance, one report noted that short periods of fasting were effective and well-tolerated. Patients experienced a marked sense of well-being in addition to losing about 2.5 lbs in body weight per day (Bloom, 1959). Based on this, another study employed fasts ranging from one to fifteen days for reducing obesity in diabetic and non-diabetic patients. The study gradually moved to one and two-day fasts at varied intervals to allow for continued weight reduction and maintenance. The study concluded that fasts of four to fourteen days are an effective way of reducing obesity (Duncan, 1963).

Historically, studies have focused on complete starvation diets and those incorporating low-calorie intake. Starvation therapy led to successful weight loss. But the costs were high, and not just in terms of money. The patients had to be in the hospital throughout the starvation period to ensure compliance and for the sake of their own safety. Essential nutrient depletion and electrolyte imbalance were common side effects. However, most of these were reversed upon returning to a normal diet. There were psychological implications for the patients who reported a loss of body weight, which was actually water weight loss. Low-calorie diets were marked as safer and equally effective if based on low-carbohydrate intake (Howard, 1975).

While the term has been around for ages, it was popularized in 2012 by Dr. Michael Mosley's television documentary "Eat Fast, Live Longer" and his book, *The Fast Diet*. In the documentary, he put himself through a succession of a four-day fast, an alternate day fast, and a two-day fast to test the theory behind intermittent fasting. *The Fast Diet* was a book focused entirely on the 5:2 diet approach, which we will cover later in this book. Subsequently, Kate Harrison generated positive buzz when she spoke of her own experiences with the 5:2 diet. In 2016, Dr. Jason Fung made the concept of intermittent fasting more doable when he self-experimented it, going up to three-week-long fasts. It is notable that on his second attempt, he gave himself 18–20 hour gaps between eating and felt good about it. He went on to popularize methods of intermittent fasting in literature, including success stories of his patients and elucidating the science behind the practice.

Unfortunately, there is a marked lack of theoretical terminology to define different intermittent fasting programs. One definition views it from an umbrella perspective as, "recurring eating patterns wherein individuals go for extended periods of time, between 16–48 hours, with little or no intake of energy, and alternate it with intervening periods of normal food intake." Within this theory, there is a distinction between studies on frequent fasting periods that last for short bursts of time and less frequent ones which last for longer periods. They use the term "periodic fasting" to refer to fasting regimes lasting anywhere between two and twenty-one or more days. "time-restricted feeding" (TRF) is used as a subcategory of intermittent fasting to refer to an eating pattern restricted to a time of eight or lesser hours every day (Rynders et al., 2019). This is slightly problematic because time-restricted feeding is not similar to a whole day of fasting or a modified one, since these rely on the actual reduction of calories. TRF relies more on actually consuming what you would on a normal day of eating, but within a reduced time frame. The critical thing to note here is the benefits that arise from simply reducing the time frame without needing to reduce calorie intake. For our understanding, this is the crux of intermittent fasting. The focus is not on the reduction of what we consume, rather the hours within which we consume on a normal day.

As opposed to time-restricted fasting, alternate day fasting reduces energy intake anywhere between 60–100% on your fasting days. On the other days, you have free reign over what you eat and when you eat it. The most popular regimens are alternate day fasting or fasting two days per week. It is obvious why this lifestyle is appealing to dieters who would not wish to restrict calories every day. Over time, it has also been established that the periodic nature of fasting results in hunger depletion (Horne et al.,

2015). Many studies based on reducing calorie intake by a modified fasting program where you reduce intake by 25% have established hunger mitigation owing to the periodic nature of the fasts. Subjects reported an increase in hunger during the first week of the trials, followed by a consistent reduction after two weeks. In terms of physical activity, it was felt that subjects would have less energy on their fast days and would be less active. To their surprise, physical activity levels remained constant, regardless of feed or fast days. The data suggested that their subjects were able to maintain their physical activity levels, regardless of decreasing energy intake. This consistency led to regular energy expenditure on both feed and fast days, which was a key factor in weight loss (Klempel et al., 2010).

Another study establishes that intermittent fasting induces compatible cellular responses in our bodies to promote cortisol release, increase glucose regulation, and combat inflammation. During the fasting period, our body's cells engage defenses against metabolic stress and work on repairing and fixing damaged molecules. During the feeding period, this is supplemented with tissue-specific growth. While intermittent fasting shows remarkable prowess against diseases like obesity, diabetes, and neurodegenerative disorders, it doesn't work if we snack during the fasting period. We need to take our bodies to a state where the metabolic switch flips on, and the body releases ketones which fuel cells during fasting (Cabo & Mattson, 2019).

Your body constantly moves between 'fed' and 'fasted' states. This happens even if you have not begun your regime yet. You sleep for six to eight hours a day, which puts your body in a fasted state. When you are feeding, your insulin is elevated, which is a sign for your body to store extra calories in your fat cells. When this happens, your body stops burning fat and takes to burning glucose (energy from your last meal) instead. When you are in the fasted state, your insulin is low and insulin opposing hormones like glucagon are in elevation. This signals your body to burn stored body fat from fat cells, thereby allowing you to burn fat instead of glucose for energy. Simply speaking, your body can only burn stored fat when fasting and store fat when fed (Naiman & Shewfelt, 2020). The fed state begins when you start eating, and it takes your body the next few hours to digest and absorb your meals. This causes a spike in insulin, which shuts off fat loss. After about three to five hours, your body enters the post-absorptive stage, which lasts anywhere between eight and twelve hours. This is the stage after your last meal, once you have begun fasting. In the fasted state, the previously inaccessible fat becomes available for burning. Our bodies do not enter this stage until twelve hours after our last meal, so it is crucial to keep this in mind when we commence this journey. Many of us are not aware of this when we begin our regimens and because of this, we burn out far before we reach the fat-burning state of being. This is key to weight loss in intermittent fasting and time-restricted feeding. If you are practicing the latter, the underlying philosophy of losing weight irrespective of what you are eating, how much you are eating, and how often you are exercising will hold true only if you allow your body to enter the fasted stage.

At this stage, you have established an understanding of both intermittent fasting and time-restricted feeding. Regardless of which one sounds more lucrative, go with a plan that suits your state of well-being. The core of the two systems is training your body to adapt to a disciplined lifestyle. When you begin a regime, your first instinct will be to consider it too difficult. You may look for immediate changes, hate the initial fatigue and hunger, and want to return to where you began. At each point, remind yourself of why you began in the first place. If you have opened this book after years of failed crash diets, you know that short-term activities only provide short-term results. This is a commitment to your body to do and be better.

Before you begin your journey, consult with a doctor and a dietician. Do not begin something simply because you find it lucrative. No human body is made the same way; every atom has its own idiosyncrasies. When we go to a restaurant, we always ask for a menu before ordering. We choose something befitting our pallet and liking. In the same way, before you begin intermittent fasting, find the right fit.

Once you have the approval of your doctor, you can chart out a plan for yourself. You can take up the daily fasting approach, where you restrict eating within six to eight hours every day. An example is the 16/8 approach to fasting, where you fit your calorie intake within eight hours and fast for sixteen. This is an example of time-restricted feeding. Another approach is the 5:2 method, where you eat regular meals five days a week. On the other two days, you partake in a very limited calorie diet ranging between 600-800 kcal. You may choose to do the two fasting days one after the other or stretch them out over the week. In the latter case, you could restrict on, say, Tuesdays and Thursdays, and eat normally on the other days. Alternatively, there is a 20-hour fast day, which is also a practice in some religions. During such fasts, you end with a big meal after the fasting period is over. There is an overnight fast, which goes up to 14 hours. This is beneficial for people with low hunger tolerance since a significant part of the fasting period is spent asleep. There is alternate day fasting, where you eat regularly one day and reduce your intake to 20 percent of that on the next, and repeat this pattern consistently (Schwartz, 2018). We will discuss these in detail soon.

If you are considering going long periods without food, say anywhere between 36–72 hours, please be aware that this comes with a host of negative health impacts. You will be exhausted and anxious, and you may experience vertigo, body imbalance, and dehydration. Another side effect—your body may start storing more fat in response to a longer fast. We have reached this stage in evolution from when we were nomads and hunter-gatherers. Our ancestors had to go for long periods without food and because of this, part of our system goes into emergency mode when left without nourishment for too long. When you go into this stage of depletion, you are warning your body that something is wrong and it has to hold on even more tightly to accumulated fat (Intermittent Fasting: What Is It, and How Does It Work?, n.d.). Hopkins neuroscientist Mark Mattson verifies that two to four weeks of crankiness are normal before your body adjusts to your new routine. He also notes that those who make it through this period stick with the plan. Success is best felt when it is long-term.

An added advantage of time-restricted eating is that you don't have to crave forbidden foods. Nothing is restricted so long as it is eaten within your prescribed time frame. This is one reason why people prefer the 16:8 approach over the 5:2 one. The latter increases cravings, therefore becoming harder to keep up with. You will also have to adjust according to your social setting. People may judge you for your food choices and why you are not partaking in eating at social gatherings. When you make this commitment, you have to understand that your body comes first. Our minds are programmed to enjoy a form of routine and structure, and when you fall into this pattern, it will become a way of life for you.

Chapter 2: Alexa, What Does the Internet Say?

The worldwide technological boom has, in some ways, accounted for the increase in health problems. Things are easily accessible, food is available cooked and stored in packets, and films are just seconds away in your smartphone channel subscriptions. Entertainment has become less about playing outdoors and more focused on simulated worlds in video games. The consumer culture is a major detriment when it comes to a healthy lifestyle. Individuals are far more reliant upon computers and technology to get by with their daily living. However, technology also has a positive role to play in terms of helping people become aware of better ways to manage their health (Gilmore et al., 2014).

Dr. Jason Fung is an established nephrologist based in Toronto. He is also an expert in intermittent fasting and low-carbohydrate diets. He runs a successful website called *The Fasting Method.* If you visit his page, you will encounter a structured guideline with nearly everything to help you get started. He gives you a simple explanation of the science of fasting as being alternate cycles of fasting and eating. He goes on to note that since 2010, the number of hits for "intermittent fasting" has gone up over 10,000%, owing to its propensity in helping weight loss and reversing the effects of type 2 diabetes. *The Fasting Method* asks us to look at our bodies as a sugar bowl. If we keep on piling more sugar than we take out of the bowl, it will spill out and enter the surrounding areas, which in this case is the blood. And that's type 2 diabetes. When you are entering a fasted state, you are allowing your body the chance to burn off the glucose that is being stored in your cells as fat. Dr. Fung's website publishes a regular blog, addressing issues such as muscle loss during fasting and fasting's contribution to growth hormones and offers a fully personalized program for people looking for a place to begin (Fung, 2020).

While *The Fasting Method* is a web page solely focused on, well, just that; other channels are offering a plethora of educational information on the topic. James Clear, who you may know as the author of *Atomic Habits*, has a page on his blog dedicated to understanding the magic behind intermittent fasting. He begins persuasively, calling intermittent fasting a "pattern of eating, not a diet." If I am to take this one step further, I would say that intermittent fasting is more than this; it is a way of life. But we shall come to that eventually. Clear describes intermittent fasting as a kind of meal schedule that will help you lose weight and get fit while you eat. Many of us feel controlled by our eating habits. Intermittent fasting is a way to control them instead. It is empowering. His definition is more consistent with time-restricted feeding because he subsequently says that intermittent fasting doesn't change the what of your eating, simply the when of it. He goes on to describe a few styles of fasting that you can incorporate, the benefits of each, and how you can adapt fasting to your life so that the results are meaningful and long-lasting (Clear, n.d.).

I'm sure, by now, all of us are familiar with YouTube. Many of you may also be familiar with Ted Talks, an American media organization that posts meaningful discussions online. Fasting is a topic covered in a number of these discussions. For instance, the Ted Talk of Cynthia Thurlow, a functional nutritionist, in Greenville on May 16, 2019, is all about the transformational nature of intermittent fasting. She begins with the catchline, *"What if I told you that breakfast being the most important meal of the day was wrong?"* She debunks the whole notion of multiple meals, noting the escalating rates of obesity, diabetes, and cardiovascular diseases. The concept of "calories in, calories out" has had negative health impacts on most of her female patients. Many women have been conditioned to accept weight gain as a natural outcome of aging. Thurlow disagrees. Eating all day long (a diet fad in some cases) is the reason so many of us are struggling with health issues. Practicing this trend exhausts our pancreas and the whole digestive system, preventing normal functioning. Thurlow discusses the difference between sugar and fat burners. The former relies on excessive carbohydrate consumption and relies on glucose being burnt for energy. They are frequently hungry and exhausted. Fat burners have clear cognition, lose weight easily, sleep better, and age slowly. There are no quick fixes when it comes to sustained healthy lifestyles. Thurlow discusses the degenerative impact of eating patterns on aging, particularly in the case of female patients. My most important takeaway from this— *you do not need to be young to lose weight and be healthy.*

Intermittent fasting will help you no matter what age group you belong in. It has marked benefits for age and health maintenance the older you grow (Cynthia Thurlow, 2019, 03:15-05:21).

Other than inspirational talks and full-fledged pages devoted solely to the techniques behind intermittent fasting, there are a host of health influencers on social media channels. They practice intermittent fasting or time-restricted feeding in real-time, monitor their progress, talk you through their experiences, and give you tips on how not to get *"hangry"* (a very millennial but very correct term for when your stomach shouts at your brain and your brain decides to become furious in return).

Now, before I move on, I will pause for a minute. You have been given a wealth of information on intermittent fasting. If you visit any of the above resources, you will be presented with guidelines, time frames, diet plans, and even the ability to choose your health specialist. Before you jump into any of that, pause. This is what the resources above will never tell you— do your research before you find your fit. All of them are credible and based on sound facts. But, and I maintain this, no two human bodies are the same. Before you begin a plan, be informed about all that is required of you and everything that you can expect from it in return. We, as humans, tend to magnify everything. So, say after one week of intermittent fasting, I take a day off. The next day, I see that my weight has gone up by a few pounds. I become devastated and give up altogether.

This is not how it works. Your body is conditioned to fluctuate depending on your fluid intake, the season, the climate, and ten other factors you are probably unaware of. The key here is to feel good with the long-term goal of getting into a lifestyle that will not only make you look amazing but also have you feeling like a million dollars. Teach yourself to be patient with your expectations. The forthcoming chapters will talk about the types of intermittent fasting in detail and how they will benefit your whole way of life. Before you make your decision, take the time to understand what you are getting into in as minute details as possible.

Chapter 3: Types, Assets, Drawbacks

The key to long-term success is in the little details. By now, you may be excited to get your program and get started! Intermittent fasting is not exclusive to one type, rather it is an umbrella term of fasts, meaning that you should choose one that fits you best. When everything is said and done, it is simply an option for a healthier lifestyle, and while it may work for some, it may not for others. Choose a plan that you can incorporate into your lifestyle seamlessly so that you control it and not the other way around.

The three broadest kinds of intermittent fasting are the twice-a-week approach, alternate day fasting, and time-restricted feeding (Cleveland Clinic, 2019). The overall health implications of all of these on weight-loss, insulin sensitivity, inflammation, heart and brain health, cancer, and aging will be covered later on. For now, let us look at each of them in broad detail to understand how we can find the one that's just our type!

The Twice-a-Week Approach

The twice-a-week approach is also known as the 5:2 diet. This diet bases itself on normal eating patterns for five days a week. The other two days, you eat a restricted-calorie diet. Before you begin any fasting plan, set goals based on your body type and body mass index (BMI). The latter is an accurate projection of your weight concerning your height. Consult with your doctor when calculating your BMI, so that you have an accurate measure of your body fat. This will give your nutritionist and you an idea of your daily caloric needs. Once you know, you will be able to decide what your fasting days should look like. For example, if your daily calorie consumption is 1800 kcal, the maximum you can consume on fasting days (to lose weight) is 1300 kcals.

During these calorie-restricted days, you can make it easier for yourself by enjoying either three small meals or two big ones. It is recommended that you have a calorie-measuring tool so that you don't exceed your allowed intake. The two fasting days should be spaced out in the week so that you don't give up on the first day itself. It may take you a few fasting days to find the right plan for yourself. Good options for fasting days include lean protein such as white meat, eggs, tofu, and fish, low-sugar items, vegetables, fruit, and healthy sources of fat like nuts and nut butter.

While there are no set rules about carbohydrate and sugar consumption on fasting days, it is advisable to keep both as low as possible. This means your first preference for energy intake on your fasting days should be vegetables and lean meat, then fruit, and finally, grains. Dessert and sweet items should be completely avoided. If you enjoy sweets, consider consuming them on alternate non-fasting days. Your body will experience blood sugar spikes with increased simple carbohydrate (sugar, refined flours, and sugary cereals) consumption, which will lead to excess insulin in your bloodstream. When you follow this up with an excessively low-carbohydrate day, you train your body to develop resistance to insulin, which may become a cause for heart issues and type 2 diabetes. Be mindful of your fluid intake because dehydration is a common fallout. On your fast days, limit your fluids to water and unsweetened drinks, preferably without any dairy supplements.

As always, you must find a balance. If you are consuming 1800 calories on a non-fast day, please don't go crazy and consume only 400 on a fast day. Train your body, don't surprise it.

Practitioners of the 5:2 diet report feeling hunger signals at the beginning of their program. This makes the first few weeks of adjustment hard. But they also state that they found it doable and effective in the long run. For some, the diet became an opportunity to improve physical activity and metabolic health. This indicates positive hormonal-metabolic changes a few weeks into fasting. Your body's long-held energy resources become accessible by improving hormonal responses in your liver and adipose tissues. You may experience fluidity, a feeling of invigoration, and better sleep (Österlund, 2017).

The 5:2 diet comes with a host of advantages. It is flexible. You get to choose your fasting days, how you want to split your calorie intake, and what meals you want to enjoy. There are no banned food items as a whole for five days of the week, so you do not have to feel like you are constantly starving. You can eat everything you love responsibly and enjoy life while being good to your body. It becomes a lot easier to restrict on one day when you know you will wake up to a normal eating schedule on the next. Trust me, no one, not even the healthiest person in the world, can claim that they don't enjoy the occasional guilt-food. This diet allows you reasonable free reign, as long as you are responsible. Your body works wonders when it doesn't feel deprived.

On the other hand, it is human nature to begin restricting food items that will be detrimental to the regime. So, even if you are allowed to eat what you want during your non-fast days, you may begin restricting yourself at a subconscious level. For a few of us, the non-fasting days can become overwhelming. We may find ourselves consuming more calories on these days to compensate for the overall lack, making the fasting days pointless. If you have a diet that is already quite poor, making changes before you begin may be essential. So, on your non-fasting days, if you decide to fill your diet with fried and processed food items, the results will obviously not favor you. The 5:2 diet does not address exercise, which may be confusing for practitioners. You may find physical mobility difficult on fasting days and face slight headaches. While the overall benefits of the diet are remarkable, you must consider these limitations.

The Alternate Day Fast

This diet plan follows the 'feast-fast' cycle. As the dieter, you switch feeding days with fasting ones. The alternate day fast is slightly different from the 5:2 diet. The latter lets you choose your fast days. The former makes you alternate one feeding day with a fasting day.

This is supposed to flip your metabolic switch, thereby enabling your body to burn fat instead of glucose for energy. According to Krista Varady (a professor of nutrition at University of Illinois, Chicago), deprivation does not work. When you refuse your body from fulfilling a craving, it will succumb sooner or later. The alternate day fast suggested by her restricts calorie intake to 500 kcal every other day. This is the fasting part of it. On feasting days, you can eat as much as you like. The premise to this is simple—keep your body guessing (Varady & Gottlieb, 2014). When you reduce your calorie intake every day, keeping it at a consistently low level, your body catches on pretty quickly. And to the body, this is a warning signal that you are starving. When this happens, rather than burning fat, it becomes more intent on conserving fat stores for survival. Know those unhealthy love stories where the protagonist cannot seem to let go of the anti-hero? Yes, that's exactly what happens.

On the fast days, your food intake should include 50 grams of lean protein, vegetables, and a healthy amount of water or low-calorie fluids. Coconut water is a great way to keep those electrolytes running. Black coffee, cucumber juice, watermelon juice, and liquor teas are also good options. For vegetarians, measure out a cup of lentils and remember that lentils can be quite dense in calories if you are not careful. A cup worth contains about 18 grams of protein. One gram equals four calories, and this should be a good place for you to begin. The idea is to reduce the number of calories required to maintain your current weight by 50–75%.

On the feed days, you can eat what you want and maintain your normal caloric intake. Varady suggests that you can even go above it (Varady & Gottlieb, 2014). The body, according to her studies, is becoming trained to use the calories you consume to burn fat and keep your metabolism up while maintaining an overall weekly deficit. Look at the math behind this. Say you are a person whose daily calorie consumption is 2000 kcal. On your fast days (three days) you consume 1000 kcal each. That amounts to 3000 kcal for the week. On your feast days, you consume 2000 for three days and 3000 for one. That totals 9000 kcal. So, your weekly consumption is 12,000 kcal. If you were to consume 2000 each day, your weekly consumption would be 14,000 kcal. And there we have it, the holy deficit.

The obvious advantage is that you will lose weight if that is your goal. When you lose weight, other health benefits follow. A study where participants alternated thirty-six hours of zero-calorie intake with twelve hours of unrestricted eating (please do not try this without medical supervision) shows that they consumed 35% fewer calories, losing about 7.7 lbs in a month. They continued to burn fat for fuel, even on their feasting days. Their bodies showed a marked reduction in levels of sICAM-1, a contributing factor of age-related diseases and inflammation (Stekovic et al., 2019). This kind of fasting was also shown to increase longevity, lower levels of cholesterol, and promote heart and liver health (Rozing et al., 2010). Alternate day fasts also allow your body to replace old, depleted cells with new ones, the term for which is Autophagy.

However, this diet is not easy for everyone to follow. It is far more extreme than the other types of intermittent fasting in that, on your fast days, you are in a restrictive diet zone. For those of us who get discouraged by the toughness of an approach, this may not be the best method to pick up. All intermittent fasting approaches come with disclaimers on who should not practice them. We will get into that a little later, but for now, simply judge yourself on your motivation. If you are looking for something a little easier, study the other approaches. This diet also makes some people go overboard on the feasting days, and the overall effect is ruined. Your resilience will be tested by this approach, so consider where your willpower levels before you begin.

Time-Restricted Feeding

Time-restricted eating consolidates your calorie intake within a 6–10 hour time frame every day, without any other changes to your diet. This means that within the 6–10 hour window, you consume your calories as you normally would and once that window is over, you do not consume anything except water and zero-calorie liquids. The median duration of eating is shown to be 14.5 hours every day, debunking the assumption that most of us go through a fast when we are asleep (Gill & Panda, 2015). When it comes to weight loss, eating "around the clock" may be a reason why so many of us are unsuccessful (Rynders et al., 2019). While limiting calories may also help when you are limiting the duration, it is not a prerequisite of this approach.

Time-restricted eating reduces body weight, improves tolerance to glucose, acts as a shield against hepatosteatosis (fatty liver disease), improves overall metabolic flexibility, and has benefits for good gut function and heart health (Regmi & Heilbronn, 2020).

Researchers noted the potential benefits of time-restricted eating in a study involving 19 patients with metabolic complications like obesity, elevated blood pressure, and hyperglycemia. The patients were selected for a 12-week intervention. On each day, they had a 10-hour window to consume their calories and log intake. They wore activity and glucose monitors for two weeks to track expenditure (outside the fast) and intestinal glucose levels. At the end of the study, results showed a loss in body weight, improvement in LDL-cholesterol levels and blood glucose values, and reduced blood pressure. Additionally, the patients did not experience fatigue during the intervention (Wilkinson et al., 2020).

The potential drawback of this type of fasting, again, rests in falling willpower. It was found that, even among the study participants, patients adapted to the schedule in their own ways. Some chose to shift meal timings moderately rather than skip them entirely, and it took most of them some time to get adjusted to crunching their intake time. It is overwhelming to think that we have to finish consuming 1800–2000 calories in six hours. There's no doubting that. For some, this also means that they lose control over how much they are consuming. As always, take your limitations into account before attempting this fast. This journey that you have begun is a celebration of yourself and your willpower.

I'm going to pause for a minute and talk about our body's unique ability to adapt to fat. Humans can fuel themselves with stored body fat instead of readied glucose supplies. Reaching this stage, however, takes time and patience, and your body needs to go through several stages before it can reach this one. This includes an improvement of insulin sensitivity, which will allow your body cells to use glucose effectively, thereby reducing blood sugar. It will also have to reach a stage of fat-mobilization from adipocytes (fat cells) into free fatty acids. When insulin levels are low, body fat is broken through lipolysis and burned by your liver cells. This is what we know as cell fat burning (Wolf, 2020). So, your ultimate goal should be fat-adaptation, even more than burning fat, because the former has far more long-reaching implications for your health.

Keep in mind that if glucose is available to your body, *your body will give it first preference*. Fat is more of an emergency supply. Say, for example, your city is known for floods. You have built a safe-house in case of emergencies and you store canned food items in this safe-house so that you have something to survive on should you ever need it. The premise here is not on you actually using the supplies, rather you *relying on them to get you through a period of deprivation*. In the same way, your body is programmed to store fat for when an emergency may happen. With most of us, this emergency never comes around. We become too comfortable in our lives, and the body keeps building the safe-house until it controls every aspect of our living. While you may prefer a ketogenic diet to a fast, when you are relying on keto, you are still consuming a minimal form of glucose. However, when fasting, regardless of which kind you choose, you are spending a significant amount of time without food. This necessitates your body to tap into existing energy reserves— in other words, your body fat. Intermittent fasting becomes a way of exercising your mind and training your body to exist in a fasted state where it is continually burning fat instead of sugar. Therefore, the time you spend in a fasted state is a form of exercise, a *metabolic workout*. You have to be rigid with your timings.

Another thing to always take into account is, *fat adaptation will vary from person to person*. Say you are someone highly addicted to simple carbs like bagels, pizza, sugary drinks, and the like. Your body will not reach the same stage at the same time as someone who does not like this food group as much. You will experience a harsher carbohydrate withdrawal phase, and this may last the initial two to three weeks. Any form of addiction is challenging. But with time, your body will adapt, and you will reach a stage where you will feel *better than you did when your body was addicted to carbohydrates*. At the two-month mark, your body will have adapted to your new lifestyle. It will switch to burning fat for your body's energy needs *by reflex*. You will no longer feel resistance to your diet pattern, and even if you consume carbohydrates, your body will have a far easier time switching back to burning fat when you restrict (Fledge Fitness, 2018, 03:15-05:21).

A Note on Liquid Consumption

Some of us prefer to go the water-only route when we are taking our bodies into the fasted state. This kind of fast allows zero salts, a primary water retention agent. So, without salt consumption, the body cannot hold on to water, leaving the risk of dehydration. Other fasting variations allow for salt-water, but it is difficult to consume this. Thankfully, the human body can still retain salt, even when it is not immediately available. So, if you keep your water-only fast time-bound, the need for salt will remain low and deficiency should not happen. The time will depend on your own body's requirements, so look out for when you begin to feel unusually and rapidly thirsty.

Another variant of liquid consumption accounts for juices. There are distinct disadvantages to juice consumption since they contain both sugar and calories. The results will depend on the type and the amount you consume. Natural juices will be more effective than processed ones, but all fruit juices are accompanied by high sugar concentrations, therefore limiting the scope of your fast. Green juices are a variant that allows you to drink juice made from green vegetables like kale and spinach. These are fairly low in sugar and have the advantage of good fiber content.

Your pick-me-up beverages like coffee and tea are lifesavers while you fast. You cannot, however, add dairy or non-dairy creamers to them, since this would technically fall outside the purview of a fast. All creamers come with dense calorie fortification and will not help the end goal you are working towards. Be wary of artificial sweeteners since they can negatively impact your appetite and make you hungrier. Other than this, they do not affect the dietary process.

Summing up, drink *a lot* of fluids. Don't go over what your body requires, but make sure you don't reach a point of dehydration. In the first few weeks, some of the weight you lose will be water weight. This is a natural reaction of your body to less salt consumption. When you reduce your salt intake, your body begins to release the water it was holding on to. Because of this, your weight falls, and this is a great relief from bloating. Don't lose hope if you are losing water-weight in the initial phase, because it is natural. If you stick to your regime, lasting weight loss and health benefits will follow.

Chapter 4: Weight Loss, Diabetes, and Intermittent Fasting

The quick lifestyle so many of us are exposed to today has far-reaching negative implications on our health and well-being. Obesity has become a common trend, particularly with the easy availability of junk food and lack of physical exercise. Our work and education patterns often promote a sedentary lifestyle. Restriction of daily food intake not only results in weight loss but also promotes better health outcomes, which will be the focus of this chapter. By now, you are aware of the basic advantages of intermittent fasting. With this chapter, we will begin discussing each of them in detail.

Weight Loss

An obvious advantage of intermittent fasting and time-restricted eating is the weight loss that will follow. We have discussed fat adaptation and how our body reaches the stage where it is burning fat instead of glucose for energy. Glucose and fatty acids are your body's main energy sources. Your body burns glucose for immediate energy needs, while fat is stored in adipose tissues as triglycerides. When you fast, your body breaks these triglycerides into fatty acids and glycerol, which are then used as energy sources. Your liver plays a key role in converting fatty acids to ketones, which are a source of energy for brain function when you fast. The metabolic switch from using glucose to using fatty acids and ketones causes a reduced respiratory-exchange ratio, indicating more metabolic flexibility. When your body reaches this stage, you are burning fat reserves that have been the primary reason for your weight gain. When these fat reserves are burned, weight loss follows.

A study conducted on 340 participants between 18–40 years in Saudi Arabia revealed that most participants lost weight while intermittent fasting. 87 people in this sample study lost 2–4 lbs in the first week, 25 participants lost 7–9, 14 participants lost 11–13, and 4 lost more than 13 lbs. There was an average weight loss of 7 lbs. (Almoraie et al., 2019). Another systematic review, comprising 40 studies, gave testimony to weight loss during intermittent fasting. On average, subjects lost 7–11 lbs per week (Seimon et al., 2015). Ten trials investigating appetite changes showed that there was no overall increase in levels of hunger while fasting, despite decreasing body weight.

The timing and intensity of this differ depending on the duration of your fast, whether you are eating minimally or nothing at all, and your overall lifestyle. Here's some simple math. If you weigh 110 lbs, your weight loss will not be the same as someone who weighs 190. The lesser you weigh, the more your body has to work to get to a stage of burning fat for calories— because there isn't too much of it to begin with! The key here is to listen to your body and to go at your own pace.

Insulin Sensitivity and Diabetes Control

Let me tell you an interesting story. In Okinawa, a small Japanese island in the East China Sea, the traditional population lives on a regime of intermittent fasting. It reports astonishingly low rates of diabetes mellitus and obesity. The population thrives on a local diet of sweet potatoes, vegetables, and lentils. Okinawa is one of the five blue zones of the world, boasting people who live exceptionally long and healthy lives (Buettner & Skemp, 2016). Similarly, members of the Calorie Restriction Society, a not-for-profit that aims to educate people to live better and longer, report low rates of diabetes, good insulin sensitivity, and little inflammation or oxidative stress. They follow a method of calorie restriction that allows for optimum nutrition. All the studies showed tremendous improvement in insulin sensitivity (Barnosky et al., 2014).

The problem with obesity is that the underlying cause is often hormonal and related to our genes, not so much the result of a caloric imbalance. Insulin is your body's fat-storing hormone. When eating, the levels of insulin in our bodies increase, and this is a signal for our bodies to store some energy in the form of fat for later consumption. This was potentially useful thousands of years ago when famine and starvation necessitated long periods without food. But in the current age, excessive levels of insulin are a natural cause of obesity as we do not face famines anymore.

So, this naturally means that to reduce weight and fight obesity, and subsequently diabetes, we need to strike a balance when it comes to insulin production. Too much insulin will keep signaling your body to store energy as fat. And, if your body cannot use the insulin that is being produced, the result is type 2 diabetes.

Insulin is your body's magic potion. It helps your body control sugar levels by signaling your liver, muscles, and fat cells to use glucose in your blood for energy. When your insulin sensitivity is low, you develop insulin resistance. Your body cells cannot absorb as much glucose, which means that there is much more sugar in your body. Without insulin, this sugar will not be burnt. So, you end up with excess blood sugar, which, if uncontrolled, progresses to type 2 diabetes. People with diabetes mellitus not only have trouble with reduced cell response to insulin, but they also suffer from poor pancreatic function.

Your pancreas is your insulin-producing organ. Those with diabetes typically cannot access enough to control the movement of sugar in their blood. This leads to a host of cardiovascular and physiological issues the older you grow. If you get diabetes, your body will not be able to use the insulin efficiently. So, while it will be produced, it will not be used. It will keep acting as an enabler for fat storage. *In type 2 diabetes, blood sugar levels rise high not because of your body's inability to produce insulin, rather its inability to use it.*

A study conducted at the Pennington Biomedical Research Center based its findings on 8 pre-diabetic men. It was found that those who engaged in time-restricted eating and finished their meals by mid-afternoon within eight hours had increased insulin sensitivity and a better pancreatic response to blood glucose. This was in comparison to a group that consumed their meals over 12 hours, although both groups were consuming the same number of calories (Sutton et al., 2018). This effectively means that intermittent fasting may help the cells use up blood sugar faster and increase pancreatic responses to rising blood sugar levels. When you are fasting, your body's first response will be to use up the glucose content. Once the glucose reserves are used up, it will move on to burning fat for energy. After the 8–12 hour window, the potential for extra glucose in your blood automatically reduces, which comes with the added benefit of increased insulin sensitivity.

The direct relationship of intermittent fasting with diabetes prevention is subtle. When you begin a program that is meant to benefit your body, all your organs benefit from it as a whole. Imagine yourself as a driver on a road-trip who has been behind the wheel for ten hours straight. The more you keep driving, the more tired you feel. This is a natural course of events of your body responding to stress and overexertion. Too many of us have subscribed to a millennial lifestyle where work is sedentary and food is instant. On the other hand, both contribute to an increased amount of stress. Imagine you are tending to a garden and you keep watering it for 14 hours a day. Will the plants survive? Similarly, your body is a living organism in need of upkeep. When you engage in a period of fasting, you are allowing your body's internal organs to work more and to actually engage in using up your reserves, rather than just wait for a fresh calorie dump.

Dr. Jason Fung is a household name when it comes to intermittent fasting. His work on the topic is legendary, and what is notable are the success stories of his patients. In one such story, one of his patients speaks of the miraculous effects of intermittent fasting on her overall health. After being diagnosed with type 2 diabetes, she was left with little choice. However, when she turned to intermittent fasting and eating healthy, she found her health improving. Her chronic yeast infections, bacterial infections, the tingling of her fingers, muscle burn, and spasms— all of these eventually disappeared. Additionally, her hormonal imbalances were also addressed (Fung & Moore, 2016).

I will end with a word of caution. While insulin sensitivity is shown to benefit from intermittent fasting, do not engage in the latter without prior consultation and advice from a physician. Long periods of fasting with diabetes can cause hypoglycemia, where your blood sugar levels fall alarmingly low, causing dizziness, disorientation, headaches, and a significant drop in energy. I cannot stress this enough— find your method. Research, study, and then study some more. Practice, when based on sound research, is far more likely to help you succeed.

Chapter 5: Autophagy and Cancer

Our body's cells manufacture components for proper function. Similarly, they must also break down damaged and unnecessary organelles to maintain a balance. For this, cells use two pathways for degradation. The first is the proteasome, which breaks down short-lived proteins. The second is autophagy, which is induced by limiting nutrients and cell stress. Autophagy degrades most long-lived proteins, protein aggregates, and decaying organelles. It allows for cells to survive stress generated from the exterior environment and internal stresses, like damaged organelle accumulation and pathogen invasion. It promotes homeostasis (a healthy cellular function state), tissue remodeling, growth control, and overall cellular rejuvenation (Legakis & Klionsky, 2006).

In essence, autophagy is a way for your body to replace damaged cells with new, healthy ones. The literal meaning of the term is "eating of the self." As a process of self-denudation, it helps balance sources of energy during development and periods of nutritional stress. It plays the role of your body's housekeeper, removing malfunctioning proteins, damaged organelles like endoplasmic reticulum, and cytosolic (intracellular) pathogens. Additionally, it has been linked with clearing senescent cells, which are cells that have grown too old and exist in tissues but do not die. Autophagy protects against genome instability, which refers to high-frequency mutations in a cellular lineage genome. This translates to protection against cancer, neurodegeneration, autoimmune diseases, and liver problems (Glick et al., 2010). We further classify autophagy as general or selective. The former packages cytoplasm and delivers them to lysosomes for degradation. It is selective autophagy that targets the damaged cell components.

So, in response to stress, autophagy attacks damaged proteins and cells and drives them out. It can prevent the spread of cells with cancer mutations and also limit genomic cell mutation. By enabling senescence, it can limit genomic instability, which in turn prevents the growth and progression of tumors and limits the spread of oncogenic mutation. The result is a suppression of tumorigenesis. It helps homeostasis and helps maintain a stable, healthy body environment by eliminating unnecessary components and regulating metabolism. If your body is not engaged in autophagy, the persistence of old and damaged components can lead to inflammation and a cancer-prone environment (Chen & White, 2011). In a state of cancer, your cells keep dividing, taking up unavailable space in your body, and destroying body tissues.

While autophagy is a natural occurrence within the human body, it is believed that there are triggers that induce it to work better. Intermittent fasting is considered to be one of them. When you fast, your body goes without food for long periods. This is different from calorie restriction, where you are reducing calories but not manipulating your feeding hours. Fasting may incorporate calorie restriction, but it does not have to. During fasted periods, the glucose levels in your body are already low. This means insulin is also low, which triggers glucagon, the body's blood sugar-stabilizing hormone. This in turn triggers the onset of autophagy. Keep in mind that in this case, you will have to go through a period of fasting long enough for your body's glucose stores to be depleted. This may take anywhere between 12–16 hours.

When your cells are in a fed state, they aren't worrying about efficiency and component recycling. They are more focused on growth and division. So, the cell genes associated with survival and proliferation are on and working. While these are turned on, genes related to burning fat, resisting stress, and repairing damage are turned off. When you are fasting, your body responds to a situation of stress by changing the way genes express themselves. At the 12-hour fasting mark, your liver begins to burn fat to release ketones. These ketone bodies activate the dormant genes, working against inflammation and excess stress. As the period of your fasting increases, your hormonal functions keep multiplying, and your cells concentrate on breaking down old components by way of new ones, therefore taking you to a state of induced autophagy. When you re-enter the feeding stage after your fast is complete, it bolsters insulin release from the pancreas and increases sensitivity. Thus, the re-feeding stage after a fast helps enhance your heart-health and cognition.

Studies in animal and human trials have shown the propensity for intermittent fasting in preventing cancer and reducing cancer growth rates. A pilot trial comprising 19 humans showed a decrease in cancer risk factors among those practicing intermittent fasting (K. A. Varady & Hellerstein, 2007).

This can be a result of decreased production of blood glucose, regeneration of the immune system by triggering stem cells, or increased production of tumor-killing ones.

In the previous chapter, I have spoken about the positive effects of fasting on diabetes and obesity control. Both of these diseases are linked to stomach cancer. Therefore, intermittent fasting, by helping you reverse obesity and type 2 diabetes progress, acts as an agent in cancer prevention. Research has also shown a positive link between a combination of fasting and chemotherapy in slowing the progression of skin and breast cancer. The combined effect of these two causes higher production of common lymphoid progenitor cells and lymphocytes capable of infiltrating tumors. The latter are white blood cells that can migrate into and kill tumors. This study also showed a positive effect of short-term intermittent fasting diets in the body's response to chemotherapy and production of stem cells (Di Biase et al., 2016).

There is also evidence to suggest that fasting can protect cancer patients from the adverse effects of radiation therapy and chemotherapy. A fast followed by a normal diet could reduce potential side effects, without leading to concerning weight loss or damaging the therapeutic process. A short study done on older cancer patients practicing short-term fasting reported lower levels of fatigue plus improved gastro-intestinal capacities, as compared to those who engaged in chemotherapy without fasting (Safdie et al., 2012).

So, in essence, fasting makes your cells work harder. Know the feeling that comes when you have been given everything? It's a kind of complacency that gets in the way of your ability to function as efficiently as you can. The same can be said for your cellular functions. While the research on linking autophagy with intermittent fasting is there, there is room for further study. Take your health and conditions (if you have any) into account, and as always, take professional advice before attempting intermittent fasting to induce autophagy.

Inflammation

Under normal circumstances, inflammation is your body's response to injured tissue. It happens when chemicals are released by this tissue and in response to this, white blood cells in your body release substances enabling cellular division and growth. This in turn helps to rebuild the injured tissue and repair the damage. When the wound has healed, the inflammation goes away by itself.

However, when the body is experiencing chronic inflammation, this process often happens even without any injury. It also does not stop when it should. In a stage of chronic inflammation, the patient will experience prolonged responses that represent changes in the cell types present at the inflammation site. This translates to a simultaneous process of repair and destruction *where it is not necessary.*

The exact causes behind this are not clear. It can be the result of failing to eliminate an internal irritant, from an autoimmune response, or by the continued presence of a chronic irritant of low intensity.

While chronic inflammation has characteristics in common with acute inflammation, the former has a different manner of response to irritants. It can be divided into non-granulomatous and granulomatous patterns, in which granuloma represents a local collection of activated macrophages (the white blood cells in your body that fight foreign substances and stimulate immunity) and their offshoots. Moreover, a case of acute inflammation lasts only a few days, which is not the case with the chronic variant (Wakefield & Kumar, 2014). With time, this process can cause DNA damage, and disrupt the proper growth and division of cells, therefore leading to tumors and cancer. For instance, chronic inflammation in the bowels can cause Crohn's disease or inflammatory bowel syndrome. This is accompanied by constant irritation, fatigue, and diarrhea. Patients with Crohn's disease are far more prone to colon cancer.

Poor eating habits contribute to chronic inflammation. Overeating increases the body's immune response. The excess deposit of macronutrients (carbohydrates, proteins, and fat) in adipose tissues causes the release of inflammatory substances from them. Excessive fatty acid deposit is a cause for oxidative stress, which causes long-term tension on mitochondria and as a result, inflammation.

Intermittent fasting may be an answer to managing this problem. Overall, it is helpful because it makes you mindful of your intake and allows your body the chance to use what is already deposited in it. It also reduces the release of pro-inflammatory cells, also called *monocytes*. The excessive presence of monocytes in the blood circulation system can cause severe tissue damage. It appears that these cells undergo a rest period when you are fasting and because of this, they are less inflammatory (*Mount Sinai Researchers Discover That Fasting Reduces Inflammation and Improves Chronic Inflammatory Diseases*, 2019).

Chapter 6: Cardiovascular Health, Brain Function, and Anti-Aging

Cardiovascular Health

By now, we have already established that intermittent fasting helps you lose weight and fight obesity. Because of this, it is linked with improving your heart health. Obesity contributes to rising cholesterol levels in your body.

There are good and bad cholesterol categories, but obesity adds to the latter and can also cause a rise in triglycerides. Some amount of triglycerides is necessary, but at high levels, it is a sign of *metabolic syndrome*. Metabolic syndrome is the sum of high blood pressure, excess blood sugar and fat around the human waist, and a fall in good cholesterol (HDL). This contributes to heart disease.

Obesity necessitates more blood to supply oxygen and nutrients around the human body, which leads to spikes in blood pressure. An increase in blood pressure is a common cause of heart attacks. Most importantly, obesity can lead to diabetes, and individuals with diabetes, as per the American Heart Association, are extremely prone to heart disease.

Intermittent fasting has positive effects on weight loss, controlling hypertension, dyslipidemia (abnormal cholesterol levels that increase the chances of heart attacks), and diabetes. It allows for the reduction of oxidative stress, optimizes your body's sleeping and waking cycles (circadian rhythm), and promotes ketogenesis (Dong et al., 2020).

In a state of oxidative stress, the body releases superoxide upon metabolizing oxygen. This unregulated release is responsible for the disruption of the balance between the free radicals in the body and other internal antioxidants. This leads to cardiomyopathy and heart attacks. A study shows that following 8 weeks of alternate day fasting, obese patients with a proclivity to asthma exhibited low inflammation levels and reduced oxidative stress. They also had higher levels of antioxidant uric acid, which counters oxidative damage (Johnson et al., 2008).

Your body's circadian rhythm dictates that all body functions occur at opportune moments, as allowed by evolutionary mandates. The circadian rhythm can be considered as your body's clock, covering your sleeping and waking patterns. Disturbance of these patterns can have negative implications for chronic heart illnesses. The heart rate and blood pressure exhibit patterns that are at their peak when we sleep. Disturbing the circadian rhythm causes an imbalance for both. The World Health Organization has criticized shift-work for this purpose. Shift-work goes against the body's circadian rhythm and can lead to coronary heart disease, sudden cardiac arrest, obesity, and type 2 diabetes (Pyle et al., 2018).

It is said that intermittent fasting enhances this optimization by helping organs like the liver coordinate with adipose and skeletal tissues. For instance, the later you have your dinner, the more you disturb your circadian rhythm. Late dinners cause increased post-meal glucose, which you do not need!

So, you go to sleep with a supply of glucose that your body doesn't need for any physical activity. This misalignment interferes with your insulin sensitivity and can eventually cause diabetes and affect heart health. Night-time eating also affects sleep quality and quantity. Intermittent fasting allows you to space out your meals so that you do not disturb your body's natural cycle.

Finally, intermittent fasting allows your body to enter into a stage of ketosis and achieve fat adaptation. By flipping the metabolic switch in your body and making it burn fat instead of glucose for energy, it necessitates healthy heart function. As a matter of fact, it may be better than a ketogenic diet that relies heavily on animal fats. Animal fats have high levels of trimethylamine N-oxide, which is associated with increased cardiovascular risks (Dong et al., 2020).

Brain Health

When you are fasting, your body will experience hunger pangs. This is because the brain stimulates the release of Ghrelin (a growth hormone) in anticipation of your next meal. This increases natural growth factors in your brain. In return, these growth factors support neuron survival and growth. You can think of neurons as information managers that use chemical signals to transmit information in different parts of the brain and between the brain and the nervous system. So, every emotion you feel is the result of your neurons and their activities.

Intermittent fasting enables metabolic switching. Your cognitive energy and brain development are at their peak stage when this switching enables the release of ketones and burning fat instead of glucose for energy. Metabolic switching opens signaling pathways promoting neural plasticity. This enables the brain's neurons to form new connections and reorganize themselves. Human learning and memory rest upon this process. Intermittent fasting also aids the brain's ability to resist injury and disease.

A paper looking at multiple clinical trials reports on the results of each of them. In one of these, older adults practicing short-term fasting showed improvement in verbal memory. A 12-month study on the effects of fasting on overweight adults facing minimal cognitive issues showed improvements in verbal memory, power of execution, and overall cognition. Another study showed significant improvements in the daily memory of individuals on a restricted diet for 2 years (Cabo & Mattson, 2019).

Take autophagy, for instance. When intermittent fasting enables autophagy, it acts as a cleansing agent by removing old and damaged cells and consequently, helps prevent neurodegenerative disorders. It also reduces brain cell damage by preventing inflammatory reactions. Mark

Mattson, a professor of Neuroscience at Johns Hopkins University, swears by the positive implications of fasting on brain health. Mattson and his team conducted an experiment on mice where they were kept in a fasted state. It was found that these mice showed a 50% rise in brain-derived neurotrophic factor (BDNF), which was induced by increases in the ketone body beta-hydroxybutyrate when fat is burned during a fast.

BDNF promotes new neuron production from stem cells, increases connections between neurons, and can even be helpful against the onset of Alzheimer's disease (Cabo & Mattson, 2019). It can be hypothesized that fasting increases the number of mitochondria in neurons, which boosts the latter's ability to form and control synapses (transmission of electric nerve impulses) and therefore boosts cognitive abilities.

There is a need for more research on how intermittent fasting is tied to improved cognitive function. For now, the knowledge that it leads to processes that promote brain health is a great place to begin with.

Anti-Aging Properties

Intermittent fasting improves longevity. Research published in Harvard University's journal *Cell Metabolism* is conclusive in stating that fasting can be the gateway to a long, healthy life. It states that fasting causes the manipulation of mitochondrial networks inside cells, which in turn increases human lifespan.

The mitochondria are organelles inside your cells. They exist in a state of fusion and fragmentation, and they are constantly changing in size and numbers through breaking apart (fission) or joining together (fusion). Both of these processes are imperative for healthy mitochondria. If you have too much of either, there will be an imbalance.

Mitochondria also play a key role in apoptosis or periodic cell death. When your body decides that a cell has become redundant, it cannot simply kill it. The cell goes through an organized disposal of its contents, which are reabsorbed and may be reused. This is important for the regulation of cell numbers in your body, and it is also a way of removing unwanted and dangerous cells. The subjects of this study were nematode worms and on subjecting them to a restricted diet, it was found that it caused genetic manipulation of a protein that could sense energy, otherwise called AMP-activated protein kinase. This is crucial for keeping mitochondrial networks in a "youthful" state of being. They also discovered that these youthful networks led to a longer lifespan, by communicating with other organelles to facilitate fat metabolism (Weir et al., 2017).

So, AMPK can be considered the key to mitochondrial processes and subsequently, longevity. When the body's energy stores are low, AMPK levels go up because it has a sensor that is triggered by a high cellular demand for energy. When AMPK goes up during high energy demand in response to low energy stores, it leads to new mitochondrial growth. This is something that leads to increased longevity.

In addition to this, fasting causes autophagy, allowing the removal of old mitochondria and the generation of new ones. It creates oxidative stress, which influences the speed at which we humans age. Stress is a response to an imbalance between free radicals and antioxidants. The latter neutralizes the harmful effect of the former and through an increase in its amounts, it has the potential of slowing down your whole aging process.

Tips to Get You Started

While these are all wonderful things to acquire for your body, be cautious of side-effects. Do not go into a program of intermittent fasting expecting to see immediate weight loss results. If you are new to the intermittent fasting world, begin with short periods of fasting. Build to longer time frames gradually. Long fasting periods, if not done carefully, can lead to dizziness, problems with orientation, and fainting spells. If you push too hard at the beginning, you may experience increased cravings. When this happens, you turn to carbohydrates and calorie-dense food the moment you break your fast, making the whole process counterproductive. In the case of fasting, as with most good things in life, slow and steady wins the race.

Choose a proper routine for yourself. So, if you read an article where it says Mr. X lost 15 pounds in a week fasting between 8 pm to 8 am and you decide to jump into the same pattern— don't. Every human body has its own functional cycle. I spoke of the circadian rhythm before, and I will mention this again— let your body's cycles decide when you should be fasting. So, if you are a night owl, don't go on a fast at 8 pm because by the time morning comes, you will be in a crash and burn stage. Likewise, if breakfast is your favorite meal of the day, enjoy it, and then plan out your fast depending on when you are comfortable with reduced/zero calorie intake.

Another thing to keep in mind is a balance in the amount of food you are eating. I would suggest consulting a certified nutritionist before you begin and coming up with a doable plan. Intermittent fasting is all about striking the balance between being given too much from the environment and knowing how to take what is just adequate from it. You have to remember that you are eating according to time, which is an external reinforcement, and not according to your body's whims. So, it often becomes difficult to not give in to temptations.

Allow yourself a treat on occasion, but don't go overboard every time your fast ends. If you go on a regular diet of fries and soda after you fast, you aren't doing your body any good. Paradoxically, this may cause a binge disorder, which is a form of eating disorder that will disrupt your body's functional patterns.

Hydrate yourself as much as you can. Intermittent fasting doesn't stretch to reducing your water intake. If you don't drink enough, your body will induce more hunger cramps, give you headaches, and may even cause nausea. Try to keep to water and avoid all sugar-based drinks during your fast. Get your caffeine kick from black tea or coffee.

Who should think twice before attempting intermittent fasting?

Anybody with high-calorie requirements should steer clear of this program. If you are underweight, trying to conceive, pregnant, or breastfeeding, this is not an advisable dietary plan for you. If you have problems with blood sugar spikes or are on prescription medication, do not attempt fasting without talking with your doctor.

For everyone below the age of 18 thinking of doing an intermittent fast, do not do so unless you have consent from and under the supervision of your parents or guardians. If you have had a history of eating disorders, be cautious. Eating disorders are often characterized by the need to be perfect and to abuse our bodies to the point where we are reduced to a dangerous love-hate relationship with eating. If there is someone in your family who is prone to or has an eating disorder, be cautious with implementing intermittent fasting.

Finally, some things you should be forewarned about—

The first few days will be extremely hard. You will notice your stomach expressing its discontent via grumbles, especially if you are used to snacking all day long. You will have to train your body to not think about food because this can trigger gastric acid release in your stomach and make you hungrier.

Some of you may already be used to mistaking food for happiness. The moment you see a slice of pizza or a burger in front of you, you think you are the happiest person in the world. For you, this period will be challenging, so always keep the big picture in mind. Keep reminding yourself of the reasons why you began.

Finally, be careful with alcohol consumption. Alcohol is laden with sugar, and it is not advisable for you in your fasted state. If you enjoy the occasional glass, incorporate it into your feeding time-period.

We've come to a stage where we can talk about some people whose lives have changed with intermittent fasting. You are now equipped with enough knowledge about how it works, what it does, and whether you should do it. If you have read through this and your answer is, "Yes, this is what I've been waiting for my whole life!" then I hope these stories, and my own will give you the final push that you need.

Chapter 7: Success Stories

In the span of writing this book, I reached out to friends and colleagues who have steadfastly believed in, well, both intermittent fasting and me. For them, intermittent fasting has been a way to reverse years of poor diets and their negative implications. I am so proud that this book has been a way of bringing their inspiration to you and I hope that reading about them will convince you of the truth of these lines by Erin Hanson:

"What if I fall?"

"Oh but my darling, what if you fly?"

Jennie Turns Her Life Around

Jennie is one of my closest friends. She is a dedicated corporate worker, the result being that she is out from seven in the morning to nine at night.

Up until two years ago, Jennie spent hours in front of computer systems, had to go on dinners with clients, and often could find no time for a self-cooked meal. She was someone who relied on quick fixes to get her through, so she would substitute a wholesome meal for readily available processed food. Before she knew it, soda, fries, and burgers became her addiction.

On December 9th, 2019, Jennie scheduled an appointment with a doctor after months of feeling weak, disoriented, and experiencing constant stomach troubles. To her dismay, her doctor told her that her blood sugar levels had gone over the recommended 10% and she should start considering insulin therapy. Jennie had been diagnosed with high blood sugar a couple of years back but had relied on *metformin* to get her through. She hated injections.

Jennie outright refused to take insulin, so the doctor prescribed *Repaglinide*, an oral medication that stimulates insulin release. However, *Repaglinide* also came with a host of side effects, like low blood sugar, weight gain, and nausea. Her doctor also insisted on another appointment within three months to monitor her blood sugar and warned her that if there was no drop, she would have to take insulin. Jennie was devastated.

If there is one thing I can credit to her, however, it is her incredible resilience in the face of hard decisions. Jennie took responsibility for her failings. She realized that the prescribed drug was not for her; it made her nauseous every day, interfering with her sleep cycle and work-life balance. She also realized how poorly she had been treating herself and that she could not remember the last time she had done something good for herself. So, she began researching how to reverse type 2 diabetes. This brought her information on metabolic diseases, the role of insulin,

insulin sensitivity, and how it could be strengthened. This is when she approached me.

I have had personal reasons to practice intermittent fasting, which I will talk about later. When Jennie approached me, I decided to put her on a time-restricted eating pattern, cut down on her carbohydrate consumption, and get her a subscription plan to a home-cooked meals company that functioned near her office and was relatively healthy. They had options for vegetables and protein and I insisted that she rely on those, at least for a month, before coming to any conclusions.

In the first week, Jennie focused on cutting down her carbohydrate consumption and getting into the fasting regimen. She found it easier to skip her breakfast and that it saved her a lot of time to go for a morning walk and to soak in nature. The first few days were hard, and at about nine in the morning, she would get cranky and call me up with the express intention of screaming at me. However, she stuck with it and after seven days, it wasn't so hard anymore. She began her fast at 10 pm and broke it after 16 hours, at 2 pm. She would have a high-protein, low-carbohydrate lunch delivered.

Jennie ran on a vegetarian diet, so I asked her to substitute fries and pizza with grilled soy patties and a side of vegetables roasted with liberal seasoning and lime (so delicious!). In a few days, she began looking forward to her lunch and found that she quit taking *Repaglinide* and reduced *Metformin* consumption. Week two was also the week she experienced raising energy levels and took the time to go for longer walks. She didn't do any stringent exercise, except an hour of speed-walking between six and seven am.

In the third week, seeing how well Jennie was doing, I recommended pushing lunch to dinner. She did it with ease. So, her fasting hours increased and she took one meal a day. This was also a high-protein low-carbohydrate meal. She relied on curried legumes, grilled cottage cheese, halloumi, roasted vegetables, and fruit-based desserts. Yes, she could enjoy fruit custard and tarts two to three days a week! She also found herself appreciating her food far more than when she had been an unconscious eater. It became more valuable, something to sit down to and cherish.

After two weeks on this fast, Jennie had reached a stage of fat adaptation. Her energy levels were amazing and she could go running. The aching in her hips and calves disappeared, as did the inflammation that caused her so much heartburn. She took herself out on a date to celebrate her lifestyle in the seventh week and could eat a good helping of pasta and ice cream, of course after taking *Metformin*. She found it easy to return to her intermittent fasting lifestyle and also realized she wasn't dependent on medications on her fasting days anymore! She consulted with her doctor and other practitioners of metabolic health and reduced taking them, finally stopping altogether.

On her next scheduled visit with her doctor, Jennie found that the results of her tests were amazing. Her fasting sugar levels had come down from 7 mmol/L to 4.8 mmol/L. Her weight was down from 180 to 138 lbs with muscle development. Her waist came down from 38 inches to 34. She was overjoyed.

Jennie has been on a time-restricted eating pattern for two years. She has a whole new zest for living and a ferocious love for herself. In her own words, *"Intermittent fasting was a way to correct all the wrongs I had been doing to myself. It was a second shot at an unencumbered life. It gave me the energy to start new, appreciate food, and enjoy living, rather than just go through its functions. I feel like a million dollars, and I wouldn't have it any other way"* (J. Harrison, personal communication, February 4, 2021).

Naomi Gets Another Chance

Naomi was fit for most of her youth. She was an active dancer and she took care of her physical appearance. She was never very diet conscious, but she felt that she made up for that with her rigorous physical routine. Post marriage, however, she found herself gaining a lot of weight. She could not find the time to continue her physical activity schedules, and the new sedentary lifestyle was followed by an alarming increase in her dress sizes. A year into her marriage, she weighed 187 lbs, which was well into the obese range for her petite 5'3" frame. Her clothing sizes had jumped from Medium to Extra Large. She adapted to this change for a few months before spiraling into depression and a desire to give up on everything. This made her turn to more junk food at heavily irregular periods. Her sleep cycle was affected, and she found she had no energy to work during the day.

When Naomi approached me, I immediately realized that her condition was the result of years of poor eating habits. Regardless of physical activity, your health is influenced by eating more than you realize. At that point, she had also tried some crash diets and found all of them to not simply increase her weight in a few months, but also severely affect her immunity. I decided to put her on an intermittent fasting schedule comprising smaller windows. So, she began on a 14:10 cycle (she finished her meals in 10 hours and fasted for 14). To make this easy, I told her to begin her fast at six pm. She slept early, so with this schedule, she would spend eight hours of the fast asleep.

Naomi's diet was severely flawed. She had no portion-control and after marriage, her consumption of saturated fats, like salted butter, had increased exponentially. She also liked eating out, and a fried chicken meal was heaven on earth to her. I realized the fast would be especially hard on her given that her body was used to receiving high amounts of carbohydrates at completely unnecessary times.

So, rather than cutting them from her diet completely, I substituted with vegetables rich in good carbohydrates like potatoes and yams. For breakfast, I put her on a diet of whole wheat bread with unsweetened almond butter, half a baked potato with olive oil and liberal seasoning, one banana, an apple, and a water-poached egg. She ate this meal at 8 am. Her next meal was at noon, where she had grilled chicken, asparagus sautéed in one tablespoon of butter with lime and pepper, guava, and couscous. For her last meal at 5:30 pm, she consumed grilled fish with cottage cheese and a side of her favorite vegetables.

I made sure to keep her electrolytes in balance because going on a low-carbohydrate diet would affect this. When the body is exposed to decreasing carbohydrate intake, it begins to let go of the water it was retaining. So, in the initial phase, if someone is not careful, severe dehydration may occur. The body also needs adequate sodium, potassium, and magnesium. She took unsweetened coconut water with her breakfast daily. All her meals had a side of spinach roasted with pine nuts, paprika, and lemon.

The first few weeks were the hardest. For Naomi, it was the constant snacking that caused most of the issues. She missed the crackers and dips, the candies and sugar-laden confections, and most of all, she found that she had a lot of idle time in her hands when she wasn't constantly eating. Eating had become her hobby. She wasn't doing it to subsist, she was doing it as a way to kill time. I asked her to take up any form of exercise that she would enjoy. After some reluctance, she joined an aerobics class. Within two weeks, the Zumba routines she practiced had become her favorite time of the day.

She found herself with more energy, and most importantly, she discovered so much more to do with her life! She enrolled herself in a fitness course and decided to study nutrition to see how she could supplement her new diet more. Within two months, Naomi had dropped 21 lbs. She did not feel exhausted, the scales did not judge her, and she could see her dress sizes dropping. This motivated her to stay focused and she increased her fasting periods to 16 hours a day. In the four-month phase, her body had reached a stage of fat adaptation, and she found that even the occasional guilt-food could not stop her from her progress.

When Naomi was obese, she had several underlying health issues. Her body craved sugar constantly and if she went too long without it, she would experience debilitating headaches. Her muscles constantly ached and her knees could not carry her weight comfortably. She would sometimes lose muscle control and spasm all over. Not only were her energy levels low, but she also had no patience, was constantly in a bad mood, and could not sustain a single job.

Intermittent fasting became her answer to all her health issues. Her attention span improved, she found herself becoming more patient with everyone, and didn't feel so angry all the time. Her muscle control became better and she felt lighter and happier. At the four-month phase, she challenged herself with OMAD (one meal a day), with the idea that, if it didn't work, she would return to her previous schedule.

After six months, Naomi lost a total of 46 lbs. She gained muscle and with it, her love for dancing and activities returned. She was more aware of her body and its signals. She learned to differentiate between eating out of boredom and eating to sustain herself, and most importantly, she learned to value food. She dropped three waist sizes, felt much more comfortable in social gatherings, and her body was not her prison anymore. In her own words,

"Intermittent fasting helped me with my carbohydrate craze and taught me to control my hunger. I realized that I had been a victim of my eating habits for years! I can regulate my own needs now, and that is the most empowering thing that has ever happened to me" (N. Brown, personal communication, February 10, 2021).

57 Years Young

Leona was one of my more unusual challenges. She was someone who had tried an endless number of diets, and they had become a way of life for her. She had gone back and forth between Paleo, Atkins, and the Zone diet and spent years working through programs of instructors via Weight Watchers, Diet Center, Fit for Life, South Beach— you name it, she had tried it. However, she could not stop gaining weight. This happened even while she was on Atkins, which typically relies on extremely low carbohydrate consumption.

With the advice of her doctor, Leona tried bariatric surgery and dropped 88 lbs in the first year. However, after that, her body adapted to its new setting, and she started regaining weight. This was when she understood that the reasons for her perpetual weight gain were hormonal. She had PCOS (polycystic ovary syndrome) and it was hereditary in her family. As a result of this, her body had a naturally high insulin resistance, which meant that there was always excess insulin in her bloodstream. She realized that her problems lay not in the meals that she was consuming, but in the number of times she ate every day. Because of her spaced-out eating patterns, her body did not develop insulin sensitivity, making her store fat without her knowledge.

Leona was pushing 52 by this time, about 33 lbs overweight, and had a fasting blood sugar of 6.4 mmol/L. She was very much in the pre-diabetic state and required urgent intervention.

When Leona began intermittent fasting, she started with the 16:8 pattern. She spaced her meals out for 8 hours in the morning and began her fast at 6 pm. She decided to stop her late-night snacking, and in the first week, she found that her sleep cycle had improved. Because she implemented her fasting cycle in the evening, 8 hours of the 16 were spent in sleep, so she did not feel as hungry as she was afraid of feeling.

After two weeks on the 16:8 fast, Leona started with alternate day fasting and eventually, 36-hour fasting. She implemented the 36-hour fasts three times a week. On her feeding days, she made sure to finish her meals before 8 pm. She cut back on aspartame, turned to black tea and coffee, and supplemented her bread cravings with fiber-loaded vegetables.

Within the next few months, she dropped her 26 lbs and then some. Her fasting blood sugar fell to 5.2 mmol/L. The dark skin patches which had been a life-long effect of PCOS became lighter. At 53, she felt younger and more vibrant than ever before. Intermittent fasting gave her a solution to her acute inflammation, alleviated her aching joints, and allowed her to join a yoga class for mental development.

After years of trying and failing on different low-carbohydrate diets, Leona felt like she had been given a new lease of life. Yoga gave her another window to reach back into herself and to see how far she had come. Over the next few months, she went deeper into alternate day fasting and she even had a period where she fasted for 48 hours. She made sure to break her fasts with a nutritious liquid. We decided on coconut water, followed by fruit. Then, later in the day, she made herself a sandwich of whole wheat bread, toasted kale, and tuna seared in a tablespoon of butter with rosemary, garlic salt, and pepper. She enjoyed her meals heartily— and the best part of it, she could eat bread without gaining pounds the next second! She also took up jogging, fitness classes for older women, and became more educated on the intricacies of her own body.

Today, Leona is at a stable weight of 130 lbs, with a fasting blood sugar of 5.3 mmol/L. She enjoys vacations, can go jogging with her kids, and also loves the occasional tuna melt. She sticks to a systematic plan of alternate day fasting that she rotates every three weeks, between 24, 36, and 48-hour fasts. She says, *"I struggled with diets for the majority of my life, and now, at 57, I am in the best shape of my whole life! I may be old, but I've never felt younger or happier!"* (L. Jones, personal communication, February 12, 2021)

Chapter 8: A Day of Meals with Me!

I typically follow the 16:8 intermittent fasting plan. I begin my fast at 7 pm every evening and end it at 11 am. My meals are a brunch, a 3 pm meal, and an early dinner.

Brunch

Scrambled Eggs with avocado on toast, spinach relish, and a baked sweet potato. Estimated nutritional value: 590 kcal, 44 g protein, 54 g carbohydrate, and 20 g fat.

Ingredients:

- 2 eggs
- 1 cup spinach
- 1 sweet potato
- ½ avocado
- 1 whole-wheat toast
- 1 tablespoon lemon juice
- Olive oil for seasoning
- Fresh coriander for seasoning
- Rosemary and basil to taste
- 1 teaspoon honey
- Salt and pepper to taste

Method:

- I've found this an easy and highly nutritious meal. I scramble two eggs, making sure to include the yolk. I season them liberally with garlic salt and pepper.
- I spread half an avocado on a grilled whole-wheat toast, seasoning it with lemon and one teaspoon of olive oil.
- On a baking sheet, I place a tablespoon of olive oil and roast one sweet potato with rosemary, basil, salt, and a teaspoon of honey (delicious, trust me!).
- I garnish the avocado toast with fresh coriander, spread the eggs on top of the toast, and enjoy it with the side of potatoes.

3 pm Meal

Grilled Chicken with honey-roasted onions. Estimated nutritional value: 520 kcal, 30 g protein, 26 g carbohydrate, 28 g fat.

Ingredients:

- 1 whole chicken breast, without skin
- 2 tablespoons olive oil
- 2 sprigs of rosemary
- 1 tablespoon Garlic salt (plain garlic if you cannot source it)
- 1 tablespoon paprika
- 1 onion

- 1 tablespoon honey
- Salt and Pepper to taste

Method:

- I have a working afternoon, so I prepare this meal before-hand. It's easy and non-messy to carry around and enjoy as an office lunch.
- In a baking tray, I place a chicken breast after seasoning it with one tablespoon of paprika, garlic salt, one tablespoon of olive oil, and rosemary.
- On the same tray, I place one onion and drizzle it with one tablespoon of honey, salt, and pepper.
- After preheating the oven to 425 degrees, I bake the chicken and onion for another 20 minutes. Onions become softer the longer they cook, and when you cook them with a bit of honey, it does wonders for the smell you may otherwise not enjoy.
- I slice up the chicken and mix it with the onion, portion it into my lunchbox, and enjoy it mindfully.

Dinner

Chickpea Waffles. Estimated Nutritional value: 412 calories, 35 g protein, 24 g carbohydrate, 18 g fat.

Ingredients:

- ¾ cups chickpea flour
- ½ tsp baking soda (optional, if you want your waffles to rise)

- ½ tsp salt
- ¾ cup unsweetened yogurt (you can use Greek yogurt for a thick consistency)
- 4 large eggs
- Two tomatoes
- Olive oil for seasoning
- Dill
- Two tablespoons lemon juice
- Salt and Pepper to taste

Method:

- Dinner is my most relaxed meal for the day. It is a time when I can unwind and enjoy myself, so I make sure to eat it as mindfully as possible.
- I preheat my oven to 200 degrees, place a wire rack on a baking sheet, and place that inside the oven. I also heat a waffle iron.
- In a bowl, I mix chickpea flour, baking soda, and salt. I whisk the yogurt and eggs separately and then add them to my dry ingredients.
- I coat the waffle iron with a non-stick cooking spray and cook my waffles in batches of ¼ to ½ cups of the mix. I use the oven to keep them warm until all of them are ready.
- I like to serve this with a tomato salsa, which I make by chopping fresh tomatoes with olive oil, dill, lemon juice, salt, and pepper.

Dessert

Frozen mango dairy-free ice-cream. Estimated nutritional value: 200 kcal, protein 15 g, carbohydrate 25 g, fat 2 g.

Ingredients:

- 1 cup (165 g) frozen fruit, depending on the type you like. I prefer to let the seasons define my choices. During summer, I like to make this with frozen mango chunks.
- 1 cup almond milk. I use the unsweetened variant.
- One tablespoon honey.
- Almonds for garnishing.

Method:

- Make sure your mangoes or any other fruit is completely frozen, as this will lead to a creamy texture.
- In a high-speed blender, blend the fruit, almond milk, and honey.
- Store overnight in the freezer and serve with almonds or any other nuts of your choice.

The great thing about intermittent fasting is that it allows you to experiment with your meals as you will. There is no hard and fast diet that you have to follow and no fear of failure if you fall back from your diet plan for the day. The recipes I have provided above are simply a representation of what I eat in a day. I change my meals regularly because I like to get different nutrients in. So, while I'll have chicken one day, I'll replace it with grilled salmon the next.

On all days, I make sure to have at least five liters of water throughout. I take a cup of black coffee in the mornings and after I come home from work, and sometimes, I'll substitute regular espresso with a hazelnut flavored one.

I add a stick of cinnamon when I'm boiling water for my coffee, this helps with the bitterness and gives a mellow flavor.

I do one day in a week where I have only greens, and on this day, my favorites are roasted kale, sautéed spinach, and cauliflower rice cooked with peas and lemon. So, when you are making your diet plan before you begin your intermittent fasting program, include a variety of things so that you won't get bored. Too many of us give up on our diets simply because they become so boring after a point in time and our bodies already know what to expect. Variety truly is the spice of life; make sure to include enough of it in your diet. And as always, consult a nutritionist to know whether you need any supplements and what you should avoid.

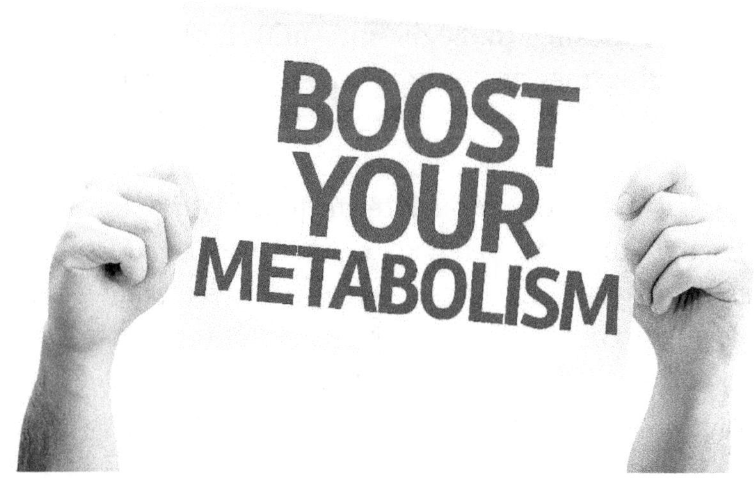

Conclusion: My Story

My dear reader, I have walked in your shoes.

When I was in my late twenties, I was diagnosed with depression, borderline personality disorder, and a host of other issues that followed. I was in a restrict-and-binge cycle, and worst of all, I had an eating disorder. I had no confidence in my body, always felt that I could be better, hated my life, and hated appearing in any social situations. At 21, my weight stood at 231 lbs, at a 5'5" frame. I was morbidly obese, I could not stick to any diet plan for longer than a month, and I was *always hungry*.

For me, choosing to begin intermittent fasting began with hunting theories online. I have always been prone to research, and by the time I was 27, I would have given anything to see some progress. This took me to pages and pages of research on intermittent fasting and time-restricted eating. It seemed worth a shot, but I had to consult a nutritionist first. Owing to my mental health issues, I also had to consider the advice of my psychiatrist. Both of them felt it would be worth trying and should it not work, we could always look for other alternatives.

I began with short fasting periods. At this point, my body was used to a college-goers diet of excessive junk, irregular meals between classes, and a lot of soda and fortified beverages. It was very hard for me. But, and I will say that to my credit, I have a very stubborn mind. At 27, I found out that I was pre-diabetic. My muscles would spasm constantly, sitting in a place for longer than two hours would cause me back pains, and I could not walk one kilometer without falling short of breath. I was at a point of either trying to change or walking straight into type 2 diabetes. *I could not let this happen. Not at 27, not ever.*

Under the supervision of my nutritionist, I began with a 16:8 fasting schedule. I think that for me, the hardest was coping with social situations. My friends would be enjoying their meals in front of me and asking me to eat, sometimes even chiding me for refusing. I would keep telling myself that there was a bigger purpose to all of this. And slowly, the more I told myself, the more I believed it.

I did not have the opportunity to cook my meals when I began fasting, but I found, to my surprise, that I could modify and experiment with what I had. In the hostel dining hall, I would rely on lentils, eggs, cooked vegetables, and take my coffee without milk or sugar. In one month, I regained control over my muscles, had better cognition in my classes, and could process what the teachers were speaking of without feeling overwhelmed. I increased my fasting period to 18 and eventually, 20 hours. In the latter phase, I would have a good lunch at noon every day and that allowed me to sustain myself. I was worried that I would not be able to keep at it, but I found that the more the days progressed, the more I enjoyed myself.

The other great thing was the lack of limitations on what I was eating. I didn't go crazy, but there were especially hard days, and I made sure to reward myself on such days. I'd have a sandwich and fries or take myself out for a nice lunch at a fancy bistro. I'd be able to resume my fast with ease and wake up with similar levels of energy.

10 months into my fast, I had dropped 66 lbs. It was astounding, and I felt like a completely different person. I was no longer pre-diabetic, I knew my body, and I knew how to keep it healthy. That itself was enormously empowering because up until then, I had been a stranger to myself. I enrolled in several nutrition courses to understand my body and moods better, and the more I studied, the more enlightened I became. I found that once I disciplined my body to eat for sustenance and to respect food, my whole thinking changed. My body responded by using what I had deposited in it for all these years, and I finally achieved the holy grail of intermittent fasting— fat adaptation.

It has been 20 years on this path for me. I am constantly learning, modifying, and educating myself and others. And today, I am here to tell you that you can do it too. If you have been shackling yourself, your progress and well-being for years, now is the time for a change. Don't think of tomorrow. Take a step today. Call the nutritionist. Make the plan. Begin from where you are, with what you have. I started when I couldn't even make food for myself. And I did just fine.

The key is to believe that you deserve a healthy, happy, long life. You have been given life as a gift, and this book is an effort to help you realize how precious it is. It has been a joy taking you through what I have learned and accompanying you until here. Now, the road is yours. Take charge of your life.

References

Almoraie, N., Alkarimi, A., & Alosaimi, R. (2019). The Effects of Intermittent Fasting on Weight Loss for Overweight and Obese Men and Woman in Saudi Arabia. International Journal of Sciences: Basic and Applied Research (IJSBAR), 46(2), 14.

Barnosky, A. R., Hoddy, K. K., Unterman, T. G., & Varady, K. A. (2014). Intermittent fasting vs daily calorie restriction for type 2 diabetes prevention: a review of human findings. Elsevier, 164(4), 302–311. https://doi.org/10.1016/j.trsl.2014.05.013

Buettner, D., & Skemp, S. (2016). Blue Zones: Lessons From the World's Longest Lived. The Annual Conference of the American College of Lifestyle Medicine. https://doi.org/10.1177/1559827616637066.

Cabo, R. de, & Mattson, M. P. (2019). Effects of Intermittent Fasting on Health, Aging, and Disease. The New England Journal of Medicine, 381, 2541–2551. https://doi.org/10.1056/NEJMra1905136

Clear, J. (n.d.). The Beginner's Guide to Intermittent Fasting. Retrieved February 27, 2021, from https://jamesclear.com/the-beginners-guide-to-intermittent-fasting

Cynthia Thurlow. (2019, May 16). Intermittent Fasting: Transformational Technique [Video]. YouTube. https://www.youtube.com/watch?v=A6Dkt7zy Imk&ab_channel=TEDxTalks

Duncan, G. G. (1963). Intermittent Fasts in the Correction and Control of Intractable Obesity. Transactions of the American Clinical and Climatological Association, 74, 121–129. https://www.ncbi.nlm. nih.gov/pubmed/14047310

Fung, J. (2020). The Fasting Method. https://the fastingmethod.com/the-science-of-intermittent-fasting/

Galani, C., & Schneider, H. (2007). Prevention and treatment of obesity with lifestyle interventions: review and meta-analysis. 52, 348–359. https:// doi.org/10.1007/s00038-007-7015-8

Ganesan, K., Habboush, Y., & Sultan, S. (2018). Intermittent Fasting: The Choice for a Healthier Lifestyle Methods. 10(7). https://doi.org/10.7759/ cureus.2947

Gill, S., & Panda, S. (2015). Clinical and Translational Report A Smartphone App Reveals Erratic Diurnal Eating Patterns in Humans that Can Be Modulated for Clinical and Translational Report A Smartphone App Reveals Erratic Diurnal Eating Patterns in Humans that Can Be Modulated for H. Cell Metabolism, 22(5), 789–798. https://doi. org/10.1016/j.cmet.2015.09.005

Gilmore, L. A., Duhé, A. F., Frost, E. A., & Redman, L. M. (2014). The Technology Boom: A New Era in Obesity Management. Journal of Diabetes Science and Technology, 8(3), 596–608. https://doi.org/10.1177/1932296814525189

Horne, B. D., Muhlestein, J. B., & Anderson, J. L. (2015). Health Effects of Intermittent Fasting: Hormesis or Harm? 464–470. https://doi.org/10.3945/ajcn.115.109553.1

Howard, A. N. (1975). Dietary Treatment of Obesity. In Obesity: Its Pathogenesis And Management (pp. 123–153).

Intermittent Fasting: What is it, and how does it work? (n.d.). Johns Hopkins Medicine. Retrieved February 27, 2021, from https://www.hopkinsmedicine.org/health/wellness-and-prevention/intermittent-fasting-what-is-it-and-how-does-it-work

Klempel, M. C., Bhutani, S., Fitzgibbon, M., Freels, S., & Varady, K. A. (2010). Dietary and physical activity adaptations to alternate day modified fasting: implications for optimal weight loss. 1–8.

Kristin, V., Gabel, K., Hoddy, K. K., Haggerty, N., Song, J., & Kroeger, C. M. (2018). Effects of 8-hour time restricted feeding on body weight and metabolic disease risk factors in obese adults: A pilot study. 4, 345–353. https://doi.org/10.3233/NHA-170036

Legakis, J. E., & Klionsky, D. J. (2006). Overview of Autophagy. In V. Deretic (Ed.), Autophagy in

Immunity and Infection: A Novel (Vol. 2, pp. 1–36). Wiley. https://doi.org/10.1002/352760880X

Naiman, T., & Shewfelt, W. (2020). Intermittent Fasting (Time-Restricted Eating). In The PE Diet (p. 330).

Österlund, T. (2017). A Personal Experience of the 5: 2 Diet. May, 6–8. https://doi.org/10.15406/aowmc. 2017.06.00169

Pyle, W. G., & Martino, T. A. (2018). Circadian rhythms influence cardiovascular disease differently in males and females: role of sex and gender. Current Opinion in Physiology, 5, 30–37.

Regmi, P., & Heilbronn, L. K. (2020). Time-Restricted Eating: Benefits , Mechanisms , and Challenges in Translation. ISCIENCE, 23(6), 101161. https://doi. org/10.1016/j.isci.2020.101161

Rozing, M. P., Westendorp, R. G. J., Craen, A. J. M. De, Frölich, M., Bastiaan, T., Beekman, M., Wijsman, C., Mooijaart, S. P., Blauw, G., & Eline, P. (2010). Low Serum Free Triiodothyronine Levels Mark Familial Longevity: The Leiden Longevity Study. 65(4), 365–368. https://doi.org/10.1093/gerona/ glp200

Rynders, C. A., Thomas, E. A., Zaman, A., Pan, Z., Catenacci, V. A., & Melanson, E. L. (2019). Effectiveness of Intermittent Fasting and Time-Restricted Feeding Compared to Continuous Energy Restriction for Weight Loss. Multidisciplinary Digital Publishing Institute, 1–23.

Schwartz, A. (2018). Intermittent Fasting. University of Maryland Medical System.

Seimon, R. V., Roekenes, J. A., Zibellini, J., Zhu, B., Gibson, A. A., Hills, A. P., Wood, R. E., King, N. A., Byrne, N. M., & Sainsbury, A. (2015). Do intermittent diets provide physiological benefits over continuous diets for weight loss? A systematic review of clinical trials. Molecular and Cellular Endocrinology, 418, 153–172. https://doi.org/10.1016/j.mce.2015.09.014

Stekovic, S., Hofer, S. J., Tripolt, N., Sourij, H., Pieber, T. R., & Madeo, F. (2019). Clinical and Translational Report Alternate Day Fasting Improves Physiological and Molecular Markers of Aging in Healthy , Non-obese Clinical and Translational Report Alternate Day Fasting Improves Physiological and Molecular Markers of Aging in Healthy ,. 462–476. https://doi.org/10.1016/j.cmet.2019.07.016

Sutton, E. F., Beyl, R., Early, K. S., Cefalu, W. T., Ravussin, E., & Peterson, C. M. (2018). Early Time-Restricted Feeding Improves Insulin Sensitivity, Blood Pressure, and Oxidative Stress Even without Weight Loss in Men with Prediabetes. Cell metabolism, 27(6), 1212–1221.e3. https://doi.org/10.1016/j.cmet.2018.04.010

Varady, K., & Gottlieb, B. (2014). The Every Other Day Diet. Yellow Kite.

Wilkinson, M. J., Manoogian, E. N. C., Zadourian, A., Navlakha, S., Panda, S., Taub, P. R., Wilkinson,

M. J., Manoogian, E. N. C., Zadourian, A., Lo, H., Fakhouri, S., & Shoghi, A. (2020). Ten-Hour Time-Restricted Eating Reduces Weight, Blood Pressure, and Atherogenic Lipids in Patients with Metabolic Syndrome. Cell Metabolism, 31(1), 92-104.e5. https://doi.org/10.1016/j.cmet.2019.11.004